The Skinny 5:2 Diet Slow Cooker Recipe Book

Skinny Slow Cooker Recipe And Menu Ideas Under 100, 200, 300 And 400 Calories

Co

Copyright

ISBN-13: 978-1482717228

Disclaimer

The information and advice in this book is intended as a guide only. Any individual should independently seek the advice of a health professional before embarking on a diet.

Contents

Introduction

Imagine a diet where you can eat whatever you want for 5 days a week and 'fast' for 2. That's what the 5:2 diet is, and it's revolutionised the way people think about dieting.

By allowing you the freedom to eat normally for MOST of the week and restrict your calorie intake for just TWO non-consecutive days a week (500 calories per day for women and 600 for men) you keep yourself motivated and remove that dreaded feeling of constantly denying yourself the food you really want to eat.

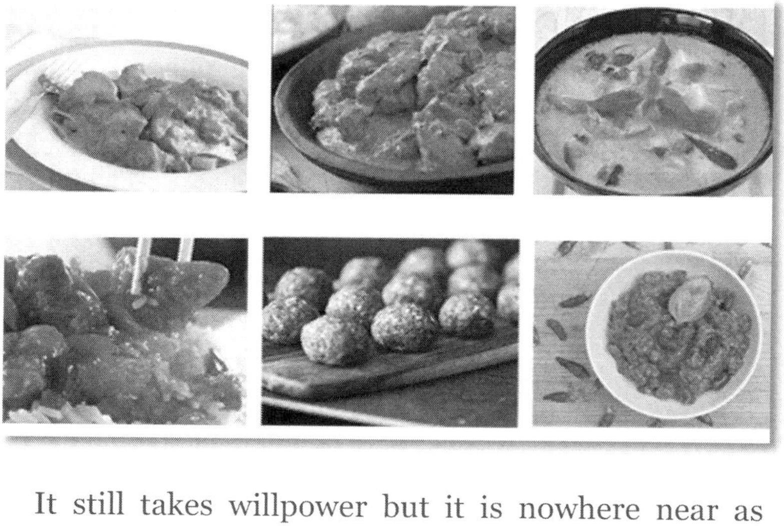

It still takes willpower but it is nowhere near as much of a grind when you know that you have tomorrow to look forward to. It's all about freedom. You choose *when* and you choose *what* you want to eat, and with the 5:2 slow cooker recipe book, 'diet' can still mean 'delicious'.

Popularised by Dr. Michael J. Mosley, the 5:2 diet plan has been adopted by both health professionals and regular people alike as a way of life which will change your relationship with dieting and weight loss. What's more, this way of eating is believed to have major health benefits which could alter your health forever.

How It Works

The concept of fasting is an ancient one and modern science is uncovering evidence that fasting can be an extremely healthy way to shed extra weight. Research has shown that it can reduce levels of IGF-1 (insulin-like growth factor 1, which leads to accelerated ageing), activate DNA repair genes and reduce blood pressure, cholesterol and glucose levels.

This book has been developed specifically to help you concentrate on the practice of 5:2, however if you want to find out more about the specific details of the science of the subject we would recommend Dr. Michael J. Mosley's work and, as with all diets, you should consider seeking advice from a health professional before starting.

What This Book Will Do For You

As bestselling Amazon authors of ***'The Skinny***

Slow Cooker Recipe Book' we noticed lots of 5:2 followers were buying our books, so we decided to put our existing recipes, along with some new ones, into easy to use menu planners to support your 5:2 efforts. We know you might still have to cook for the family whilst trying to fast, which is why our healthy slow cooker recipes will help make family mealtimes easy on your fasting days. For those of you cooking for one, you may also like to try our other book 'The Skinny 5:2 Fast Diet Meals For One'.

This book has been designed to get you through by providing detailed menu plans, recipes and snack ideas to keep you motivated and your engine stoked during your fasting days. What makes the 5:2 diet so good is that it's only a part-time diet. Because you can eat what you want for 5 days a week you will be much more likely to stick with it over time and enjoy the long term health and weight benefits.

Taking It Week By Week

The 5:2 diet can work for you whatever your lifestyle. Each week you should think carefully about which days are likely to be best suited to your fasting days and then stick with it. You can change your days each week or keep in a regular routine, whichever suits you best.

Of course, reducing your calorie intake for two days will take some getting used to and inevitably there will be hunger pangs to start with, but you'll be amazed at how quickly your body adapts to your new style of eating - and far from gorging the day after your fasting day, you'll find you simply enjoy the luxury of eating normally.

The slow cooker recipes in this book have been designed to fill you up as much as possible during your fasting days. Most recipes serve 4, so if you are cooking only for yourself freeze into meal size portions for easy use over the coming weeks. However, it's just as likely you will be cooking for everyone which is why we've made the recipes family friendly too!

Some 5:2 Tips

Avoid too much exercise on your fasting days. Eating less is likely to make you feel a little weaker, certainly to start with, so don't put the pressure on yourself to exercise.

It's better to avoid alcohol on your fasting days. Not only is alcohol packed with empty calories, it could also have a greater effect on you than usual as you have less food in your system to help absorb it.

Don't give up! Even if you find your fasting days tough to start with, stick with it - it's only for one day! Remember you can eat what you like tomorrow without having to feel guilty.

About Our Slow Cooking Recipes

The recipes in this book are simple and easy to follow, with inexpensive fresh and seasonal ingredients where possible. They are also packed full of flavour and goodness so you can enjoy maximum taste but with minimum calories.

Preparation

These fuss-free recipes are easy to prepare, and should take no more than 10-15 minutes of preparation - perfect for busy people!

All meat and vegetables should be cut into even-sized pieces unless stated. Although root vegetables can take longer to cook, generally make sure everything is bite-sized and washed before use. Remember that unlike meat, vegetables do not produce their own juices to cook in, so it's important to add the required liquid/stock to each recipe (we've covered this in each list of ingredients). Where our recipes use beans we have used canned beans for ease - dried beans are fine too but will require overnight soaking and rinsing. Meat should be trimmed with visible fat and any skin removed.

Nutrition

All of the recipes in this collection are balanced low-fat family meals which should keep you feeling full and satisfied on your fasting days. All recipes have serving suggestions; the calories noted on the recipes are **per serving** of the recipe ingredients only so bear that in mind.

Using Your Slow Cooker: A Few Things

All cooking times are a guide. Make sure you get to know your own slow cooker so that you can adjust timings accordingly.

A spray of one-cal cooking oil in the cooker before adding ingredients will help with cleaning and you can also buy slow cooker liners which make things even easier!

Be confident with your cooking. Feel free to use substitutes to suit your own taste and don't let a missing herb or spice stop you making a meal - you'll almost always be able to find something to replace it, just be careful it doesn't alter the calorie count.

Meal Planners

You will soon find out what suits you best on your fasting days by trying out all the different options. It may suit you to skip a meal altogether or you may prefer smaller more regular eats throughout your fasting day. Either way you shouldn't take in more than 500 calories (women) /600 calories (men) per day, and this includes drinks.

The menus work on a 3 week rolling basis. So every

option - whether it be leaving out lunch, skipping breakfast or having smaller meals throughout the day - has a three week plan of its own.

Not every meal planner is going to work for you and it may be unrealistic to expect you to use the slow cooker twice a day if you are out at work all day, so feel free to substitute something else for the same calories. Likewise, you may choose to prepare meals in advance so that you can stick with the planners exactly. We have also included non slow cooker snacks, bites and breakfasts to complement the slow cooker recipes and complete the plan for you. That's the beauty of this diet, you can decide how, when and what you eat as long as you stay under 500 calories(women)/600 calories (men) on your fasting days.

DAILY MEAL PLANERS

ladies first

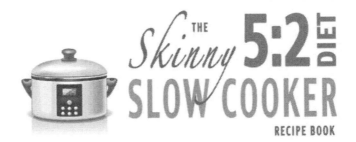

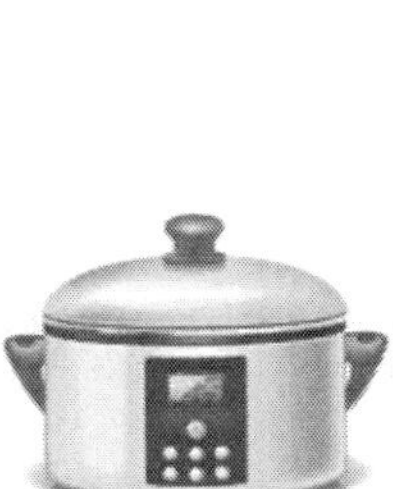

The Skinny 5:2 Diet
SLOW COOKER
RECIPE BOOK

Ladies Meal Planner (Minus Breakfast) Week One

(sc)= slow cooker recipe **(v)** =vegetarian

Ladies Meal Planner (Minus Breakfast) 500 Calories Per Fast Day **Week *One***				
	Drinks Throughout The Day	Lunch	Dinner	Cal
Day One	**Tea/Coffee/Low Cal Drinks** *No more than 50 calories*	**Corn & Potato Chowder (v)** *150 calories*	**Best Ever Chicken Curry & Cauliflower Rice (sc)** *273 calories*	473
Day Two	**Tea/Coffee/Low Cal Drinks** *No more than 50 calories*	**Bean, Rosemary & Roasted Garlic Dip & Flat Bread (v) (sc)** *188 calories*	**Tuna & Noodle Cattia (sc)** *250 calories*	488

Notes: ensure the shop-bought flatbread you have with the homemade bean dip does not exceed 100 calories

Recipe Finder:

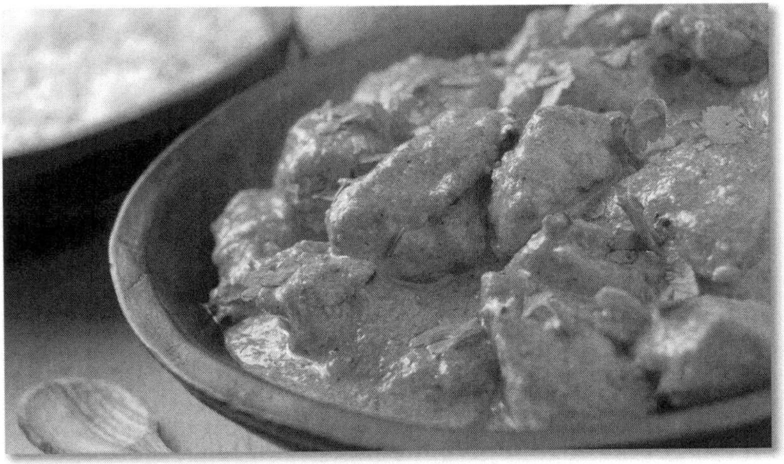

Ladies Meal Planner (Minus Breakfast) Week Two

(sc)= slow cooker recipe **(v)** =vegetarian

Ladies Meal Planner (Minus Breakfast) 500 Calories Per Fast Day **Week *Two***				
	Drinks Throughout The Day	Lunch	Dinner	Cal
Day One	**Tea/Coffee/Low Cal Drinks** *No more than 50 calories*	**Slow Spanish Tombet & Tortilla Chips (v) (sc)** *169 calories*	**Super Simple Chicken Taco Soup & 1 Low Fat Crispbread (sc)** *277 calories*	496
Day Two	**Tea/Coffee/Low Cal Drinks** *No more than 50 calories*	**Zingy Lime Chicken & 50g Green Salad (sc)** *210 calories*	**Shepherd-less Pie (v) (sc)** *250 calories*	500

Notes: The shop-bought tortilla chips should be low fat, a portion of 5 whole chips has been allowed in the calories above.

Recipe Finder:

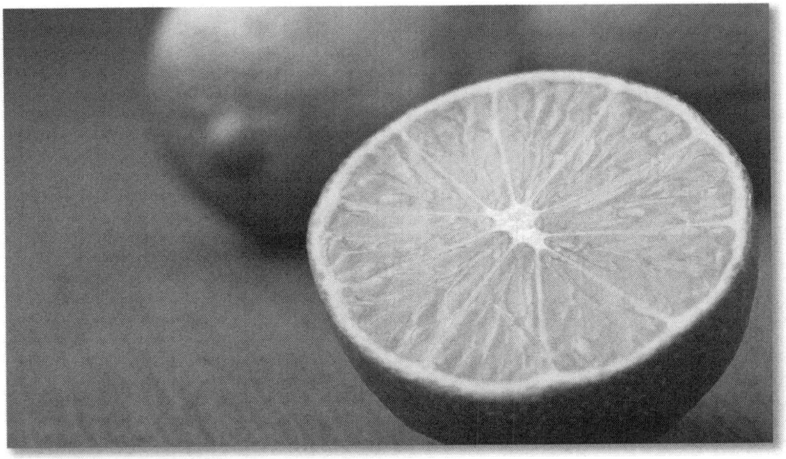

Ladies Meal Planner (Minus Breakfast) Week Three

(sc)= slow cooker recipe **(v)** =vegetarian

Ladies Meal Planner (Minus Breakfast) 500 Calories Per Fast Day **Week *Three***				
	Drinks Throughout The Day	Lunch	Dinner	Cal
Day One	**Tea/Coffee/ Low Cal Drinks** *No more than 50 calories*	**Hock Ham & Split Pea Soup (sc)** *178 calories*	**Budapest's Best Beef Goulash (sc)** *228 calories*	456
Day Two	**Tea/Coffee/ Low Cal Drinks** *No more than 50 calories*	**Asian Hot Soup (v) (sc)** *130 calories*	**Luscious Italian Chicken & 50g Salad & 100g Beansprouts (sc)** *265 calories*	445

Recipe Finder:

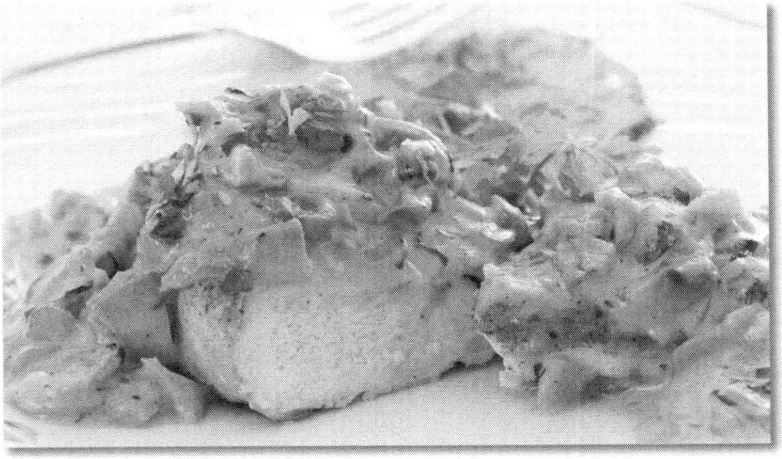

Ladies Meal Planner (Minus Lunch) Week One

(sc)= slow cooker recipe **(v)** =vegetarian

Ladies Meal Planner (Minus Lunch) 500 Calories Per Fast Day **Week *One***				
	Drinks Throughout The Day	Breakfast	Dinner	Cal
Day One	**Tea/Coffee/ Low Cal Drinks** *No more than 50 calories*	**Muesli & 125ml Skimmed Milk (v)** *170 calories*	**Sweet Asian Chicken & 100g Shirataki Noodles (sc)** *276 calories*	496
Day Two	**Tea/Coffee/ Low Cal Drinks** *No more than 50 calories*	**Strawberry & Banana Smoothie & ½ Low Cal Bagel With Low Fat Spread (v)** *160 calories*	**Sweet & Citrus Salmon & 50g Salad (sc)** *280 calories*	490

Notes: Ensure your shop-bought low calorie bagel does not exceed 100 calories per whole bagel.

Recipe Finder:

Muesli Page 114

Sweet Asian Chicken Page 56

Strawberry & Banana Smoothie Page 124

Sweet & Citrus Salmon Page 70

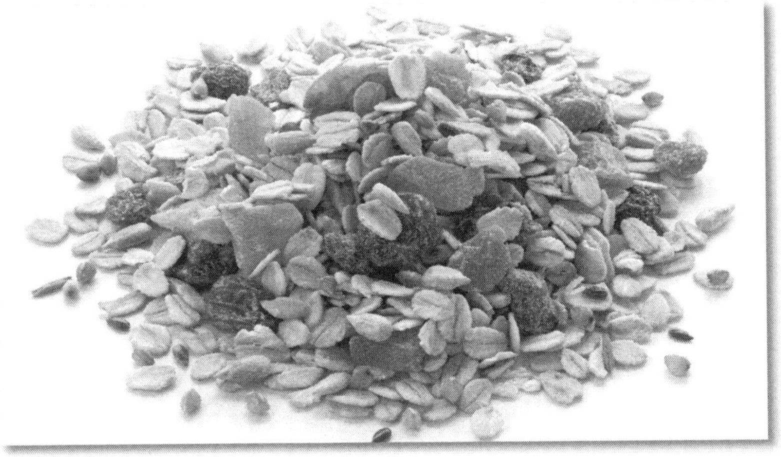

Ladies Meal Planner (Minus Lunch) Week Two

(sc)= slow cooker recipe **(v)** =vegetarian

Ladies Meal Planner (Minus Lunch) 500 Calories Per Fast Day **Week *Two***				
	Drinks Throughout The Day	Breakfast	Dinner	Cal
Day One	**Tea/Coffee/ Low Cal Drinks** *No more than 50 calories*	**Multigrain Breakfast (v)** *225 calories*	**Lovely Lemony Garlicky Chicken & 50g Green Salad (sc)** *218 calories*	493
Day Two	**Tea/Coffee/ Low Cal Drinks** *No more than 50 calories*	**Mixed Berry Smoothie & Toast With Low Fat Spread (v)** *180 calories*	**Sweet & Sour Pineapple Pork & 100g Shirataki Noodles (sc)** *258 calories*	488

Notes: Ensure your toast is less than 70 calories per slice.

Recipe Finder:

Multigrain Breakfast Page 110

Lovely Lemony Garlicky Chicken Page 90

Mixed Berry Smoothie Page 125

Sweet & Sour Pineapple Pork Page 68

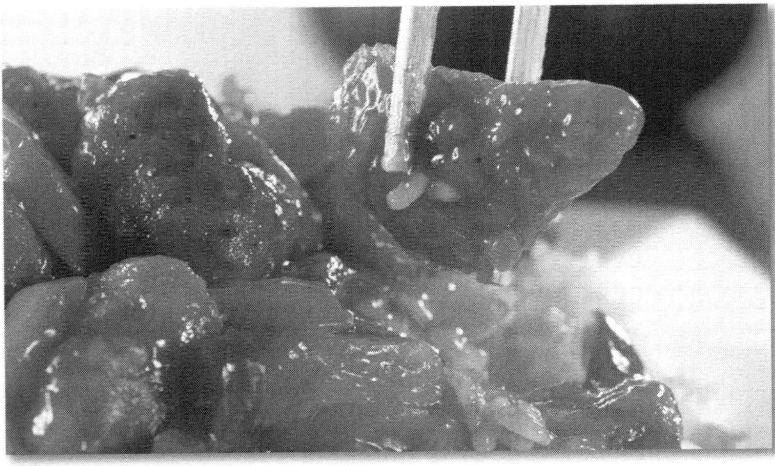

Ladies Meal Planner (Minus Lunch) Week Three

(sc)= slow cooker recipe **(v)** =vegetarian

Ladies Meal Planner (Minus Lunch) 500 Calories Per Fast Day **Week *Three***				
	Drinks Throughout The Day	Breakfast	Dinner	Cal
Day One	**Tea/Coffee/ Low Cal Drinks** *No more than 50 calories*	**Fruit Salad (v)** *138 calories*	**Lean Green Risotto & 50g Green Salad (v) (sc)** *295 calories*	483
Day Two	**Tea/Coffee/ Low Cal Drinks** *No more than 50 calories*	**2 Wholegrain Wheat Biscuit Breakfast (eg. Weetabix) & 125ml Semi Skimmed Milk (v)** *198 calories*	**Green Thai Fish Curry & Low Fat Rice Cake (sc)** *245 calories*	493

Notes: Make sure your rice cake is no more than 30 calories

Recipe Finder:

Fruit Salad Page 115

Lean Green Risotto Page 80

Green Thai Fish Curry Page 82

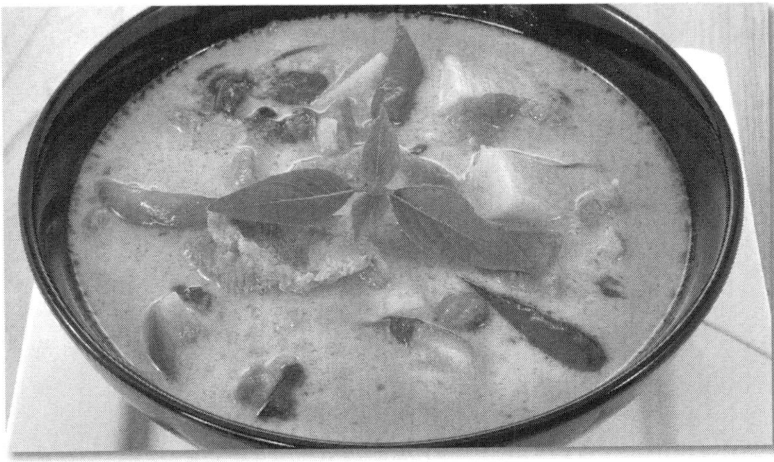

Ladies Meal Planner (Eat Little & Often) Week One

(sc)= slow cooker recipe **(v)** =vegetarian

Ladies Meal Planner (Eat Little & Often) 500 Calories Per Fast Day **Week *One***	
Day One	• **Piece Of Fresh Fruit** 90 calories • **Nacho, Bean & Onion Dip & Breadsticks (sc)** 150 calories • **Low Fat Bagel & Low Fat Spread** 110 calories • **St Patrick's Day Soup (sc)** 100 calories • **Drinks throughout the day** 50 calories *Total Calories 490*
Day Two	• **Boiled Egg & 1 Crackerbread** 110 calories • **Frozen Banana** 90 calories • **Carrot & Celery Salad** 97 calories • **Slow Cooker Baked Corn On The Cob (sc)** 145 calories • **Drinks Throughout The Day** 50 calories *Total Calories 492*

Notes: Breadsticks not to exceed 60 cal.

Ensure shop-bought bagel does not exceed 100 calories

Recipe Finder:

Nacho, Bean & Onion Dip Page 108

St Patrick's Day Soup Page 92

Carrot & Celery Salad Page 117

Slow Cooker Baked Corn On The Cob Page 91

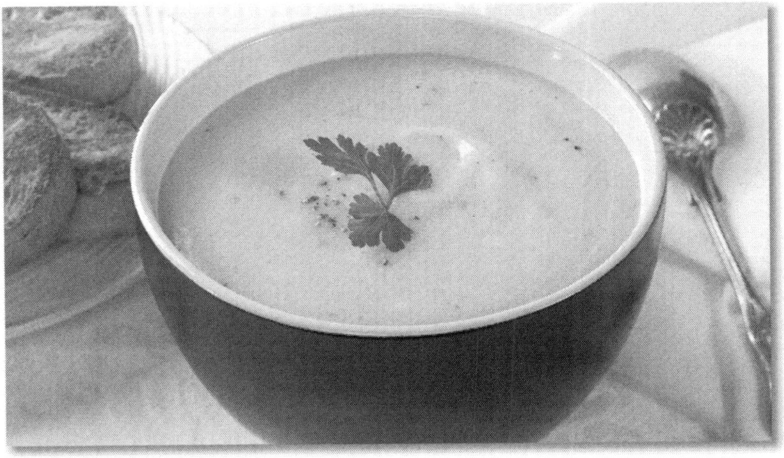

Ladies Meal Planner (Eat Little & Often) Week Two

(sc)= slow cooker recipe **(v)** =vegetarian

Ladies Meal Planner (Eat Little & Often) 500 Calories Per Fast Day **Week *Two***	
Day One	• **1 Wedge Water Melon** (1/16 of a whole water melon) 88 calories • **Corn & Potato Chowder (sc)**150 calories • **2 Dutch Crispbakes With 80g Low Fat Cottage Cheese** 120 calories • **150g Sugar Snap Peas With Sea Salt (sc)**65 calories • **Drinks Throughout The Day** 50 calories *Total Calories 473*
Day Two	• **Kiwi & Strawberry Smoothie** 100 calories • **¼ Can Tuna With Lemon & tsp Capers + 2 Low Cal Oatcakes** 100 Calories • **Hock Ham & Split Pea Soup (sc)**178 calories • **12 Plain Pitted Olives** 60 calories • **Drinks Throughout The Day** 50 calories *Total Calories 488*

Notes: Your shop-bought crispbakes should total no more than 60 calories

Recipe Finder:

Corn & Potato Chowder Page 94

Sugar Snap Peas With Sea Salt Page 120

Tuna, Lemon & Capers Page 119

Kiwi & Strawberry Smoothie Page 126

Hock Ham & Split Pea Soup Page 98

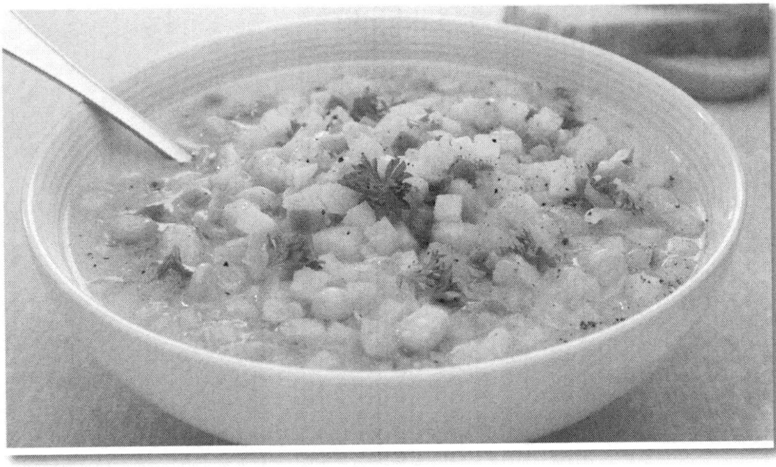

Ladies Meal Planner (Eat Little & Often) Week Three

(sc)= slow cooker recipe **(v)** =vegetarian

Ladies Meal Planner (Eat Little & Often) 500 Calories Per Fast Day **Week *Three***	
Day One	• **Slice Melon & Slice Parma Ham** 140 calories • **Small Grilled Skinless Chicken Breast With Grilled Cherry Tomatoes** 100 calories • **Handful Of Mixed Berries** 80 calories • **Slow Spanish Tombet (sc)**115 calories • **Drinks Throughout The Day** 50 calories *Total Calories 485*
Day Two	• **150g Blueberries & 1 tbsp Low Fat Yoghurt** 140 calories • **Zucchini Soup (sc)**95 calories • **100g Low Fat Baked Beans** 70 calories • **Tomato, Feta & Olive Salad** 113 calories • **Drinks Throughout The Day** 50 calories Total Calories 468

Recipe Finder:

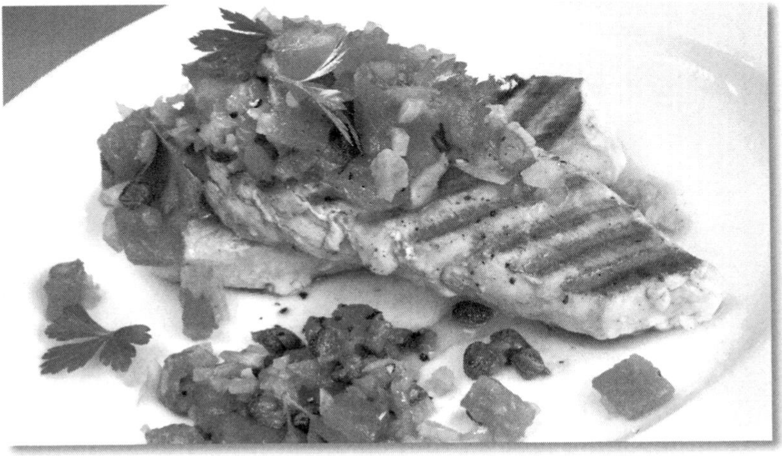

DAILY MEAL PLANERS

Men's

THE *Skinny* 5:2 DIET SLOW COOKER RECIPE BOOK

Men's Meal Planner (Minus Breakfast) Week One

(sc)= slow cooker recipe **(v)** =vegetarian

Men's Meal Planner (Minus Breakfast) 600 Calories Per Fast Day **Week *One***				
	Drinks Throughout The Day	Lunch	Dinner	Cal
Day One	**Tea/Coffee/ Low Cal Drinks** *No more than 50 calories*	**Tuna & Pita Salad** *260 calories*	**Sweet Asian Chicken & 100g Shirataki Noodles (sc)** *276 calories*	586
Day Two	**Tea/Coffee/ Low Cal Drinks** *No more than 50 calories*	**Scrambled Eggs on 1 Low Cal Toast (2 Eggs) (v)** *260 calories*	**Perfect Pulled Pork & 100g Green Salad (sc)** *282 calories*	592

Recipe Finder:

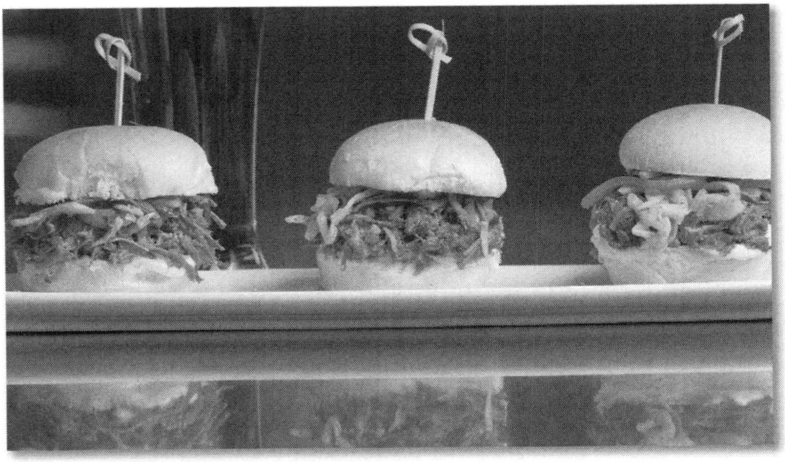

Men's Meal Planner (Minus Breakfast) Week Two

(sc)= slow cooker recipe **(v)** =vegetarian

Men's Meal Planner (Minus Breakfast) 600 Calories Per Fast Day **Week *Two***				
	Drinks Throughout The Day	Lunch	Dinner	Cal
Day One	**Tea/Coffee/ Low Cal Drinks** *No more than 50 calories*	**St Patrick's Day Soup Soup (v) (sc)** *100 calories*	**Chili Con Carne (sc)** *440 calories*	590
Day Two	**Tea/Coffee/ Low Cal Drinks** *No more than 50 calories*	**Zingy Lime Chicken & 100g Green Salad & ½ Slice Avocado (sc)** *360 calories*	**Wild Mushroom Stroganoff & 100g Shirataki Noodles (v) (sc)** *121 calories*	531

Recipe Finder:

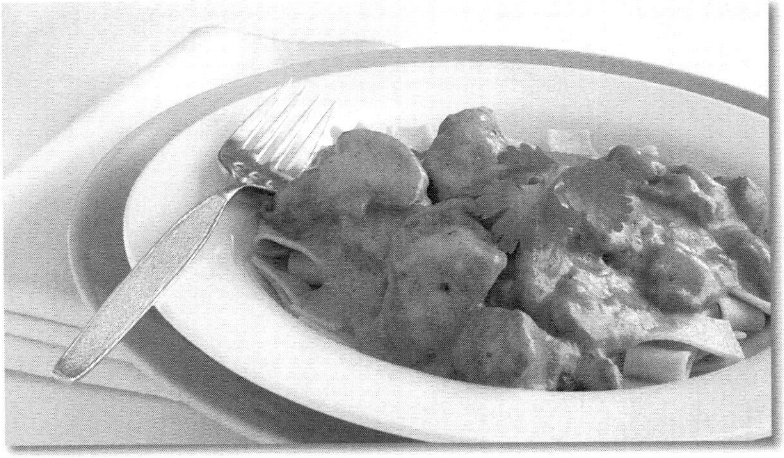

Men's Meal Planner (Minus Breakfast) Week Three

(sc)= slow cooker recipe **(v)** =vegetarian

Men's Meal Planner (Minus Breakfast) 600 Calories Per Fast Day **Week *Three***				
	Drinks Throughout The Day	Lunch	Dinner	Cal
Day One	**Tea/Coffee/ Low Cal Drinks** *No more than 50 calories*	**Corn & Potato Chowder (v) (sc)** *150 calories*	**Italian Meatballs & 100g Green Salad (sc)** *343 Calories*	543
Day Tw o	**Tea/Coffee/ Low Cal Drinks** *No more than 50 calories*	**Nacho, Bean & Onion Dip With Tortilla Chips (v) (sc)** *176 calories*	**Best Ever Chicken Curry & Cauliflower Rice (sc)** *373 calories*	599

Notes: The shop-bought tortilla chips should be low fat. A portion of 8 whole chips has been allowed in the calories above.

Recipe Finder:

Corn & Potato Chowder Page 94

Italian Meatballs Page 62

Nacho, Bean & Onion Dip Page 108

Best Ever Chicken Curry Page 72

Cauliflower Rice Page 123

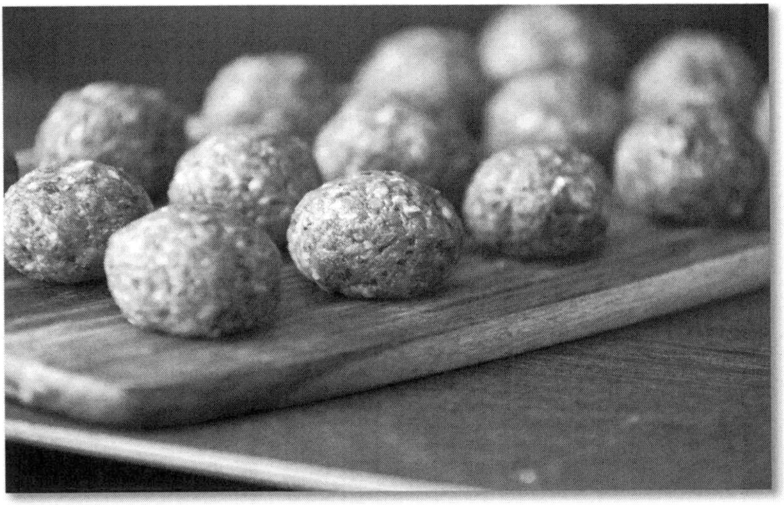

Men's Meal Planner (Minus Lunch) Week One

(sc)= slow cooker recipe **(v)** =vegetarian

Men's Meal Planner (Minus Lunch) 600 Calories Per Fast Day **Week *One***				
	Drinks Throughout The Day	Breakfast	Dinner	Cal
Day 1	**Tea/ Coffee/ Low Cal Drinks** *No more than 50 calories*	**Strawberry & Banana Smoothie & Low Cal Bagel with Low Fat Spread (v)** *220 calories*	**Budapest's Best Beef Goulash & 100g Shirataki Noodles & 100g Green Salad (sc)** *268 calories*	538
Day 2	**Tea/ Coffee/ Low Cal Drinks** *No more than 50 calories*	**Homemade Museli & 1 tsp Brown Sugar & 125ml Semi Skimmed Milk (v)** *204 calories*	**Sweet Asian Chicken with 100g Beansprouts & 200g Green Salad (sc)** *323 calories*	577

Notes: Ensure your shop-bought bagel does not exceed 100 calories per whole bagel.

Recipe Finder:

Strawberry & Banana Smoothie Page 124

Budapest's Best Beef Goulash Page 64

Muesli Page 114

Sweet Asian Chicken Page 56

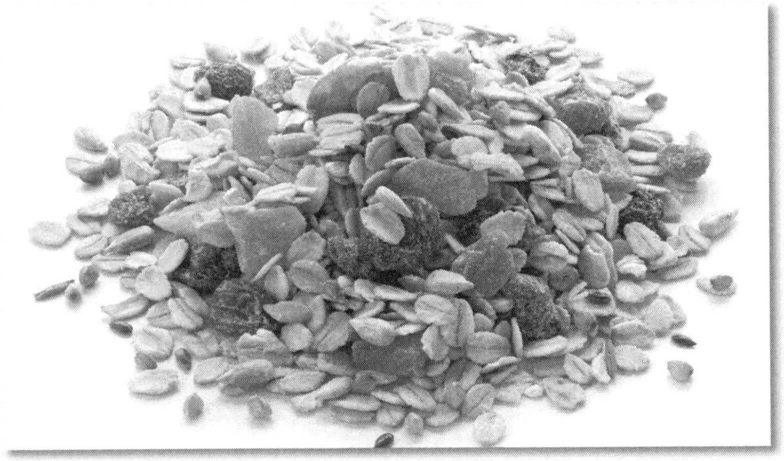

Men's Meal Planner (Minus Lunch) Week Two

(sc)= slow cooker recipe **(v)** =vegetarian

Men's Meal Planner (Minus Lunch) 600 Calories Per Fast Day **Week *Two***				
	Drinks Throughout The Day	Breakfast	Dinner	Cal
Day One	**Tea/Coffee/ Low Cal Drinks** *No more than 50 calories*	**Fruit Salad + 3 tbsp Low Fat Yoghurt (v)** *162 calories*	**Enchilada El Salvadore & 1 Low Fat Taco Shell & 100g Green Salad (sc)** *385 calories*	597
Day Two	**Tea/Coffee/ Low Cal Drinks** *No more than 50 calories*	**3 Wheat Biscuit Breakfast (eg. Weetabix) & 125ml Semi Skimmed Milk (v)** *230 calories*	**Sweet & Sour Pineapple Pork & Cauliflower Rice (sc)** *288 Calories*	568

Recipe Finder:

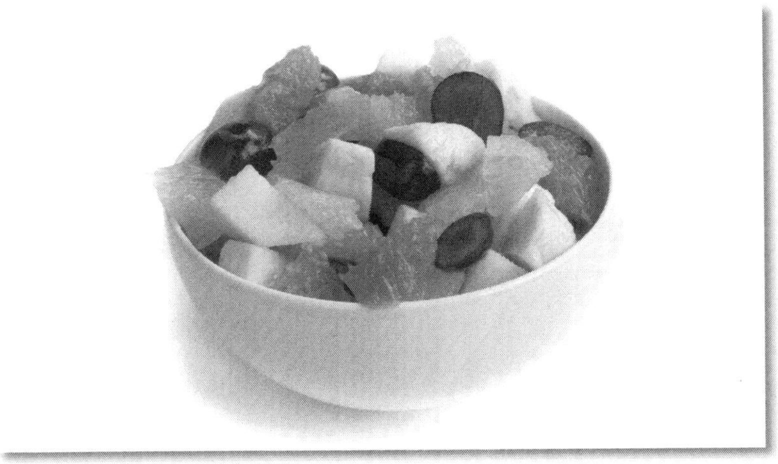

Men's Meal Planner (Minus Lunch) Week Three

(sc)= slow cooker recipe **(v)** =vegetarian

Men's Meal Planner (Minus Lunch) 600 Calories Per Fast Day **Week *Three***				
	Drinks Throughout The Day	Breakfast	Dinner	Cals
Day One	**Tea/Coffee /Low Cal Drinks** *No more than 50 calories*	**Morning Millet & tsp Brown Sugar (v)** 171 Calories	**Citrus Salmon & 90g Boiled New Potatoes & 100g Green Salad (sc)** 355 calories	576
Day Two	**Tea/Coffee /Low Cal Drinks** *No more than 50 calories*	**Mixed Berry Smoothie & Frozen Banana (v)** *190 calories*	**'Hand To Mouth' Tex Mex Tacos With 1 Low Fat Tortilla Wrap, 1 tbsp Low Fat Crème Fraiche, 100g Green Salad and 25g Grated Low Fat Cheese (v) (sc)** *340 calories*	580

Recipe Finder:

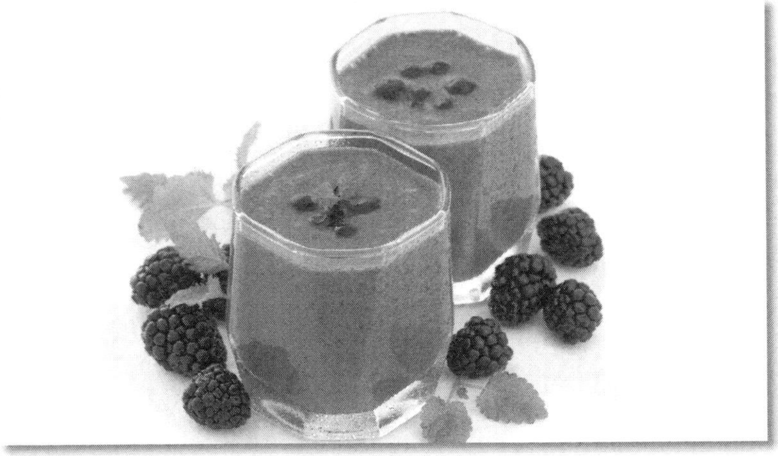

Men's Meal Planner (Eat Little And Often) Week One

(sc)= slow cooker recipe **(v)** =vegetarian

Men's Meal Planner (Eat Little & Often) 600 Calories Per Fast Day **Week *One***	
Day One	• **Piece Of Fresh Fruit** 90 calories • **Bean, Rosemary & Roasted Garlic Dip & Breadsticks (sc)** 150 calories • **Low Fat Bagel & Spread** 120 calories • **Zucchini Soup (sc)** 95 calories • **1 tbsp sunflower seeds** 90 calories • **Drinks throughout the day** 50 calories *Total Calories 595*
Day Two	• **Boiled Egg & Slice Of Low Cal Toast & Spread** 160 calories • **Frozen Banana** 90 calories • **Carrot & Celery Salad** 97 calories • **Babybel Light Cheese Portion** 43 calories • **Slow Cooker Baked Corn On The Cob (sc)**150 calories • **Drinks Throughout The Day** 50 calories *Total Calories 590*

Notes: Breadsticks should not exceed 60 calories

Ensure shop-bought bagel does not exceed 100 calories.

Shop bought bread should not exceed 60 calories.

Recipe Finder:

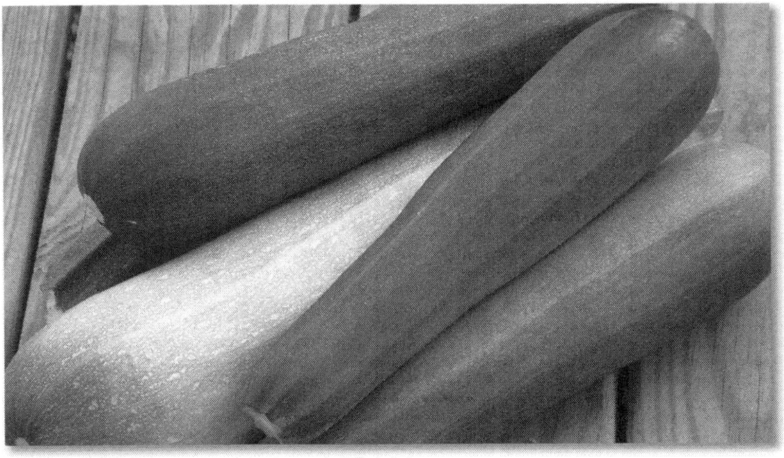

Men's Meal Planner (Eat Little And Often) Week Two

(sc)= slow cooker recipe **(v)** =vegetarian

Men's Meal Planner (Eat Little & Often) 600 Calories Per Fast Day **Week *Two***	
Day One	• **3 tbsp homemade salsa and 2 carrots cut into batons** 100 calories • **Barley & Chestnut Mushroom Soup (sc)**175 calories • **200g Shirataki Noodles With 1 tbsp Soy Sauce & Pinch Of Chili Flakes** 70 calories • **Sugar Snap Peas With Sea Salt** 65 calories • **Small apple cut in slices with 2 tsp low fat peanut butter** 100 calories • **Drinks throughout the day** 50 calories *Total Calories 560*
Day Two	• **Wild Mushroom Stroganoff (sc)** 101 calories • **30 pistachios** 127 calories • **1 Hard boiled egg** 100 calories • **½ cup /120g Non Fat Greek Yoghurt With tsp Runny Honey** 90 calories • **150g/1 Cup Strawberries With 1 tsp Brown Sugar** 110 calories • **Drinks Throughout The Day** 50 calories *Total Calories 578*

Recipe Links:

Homemade Salsa Page 121

Barley & Chestnut Mushroom Soup Page 104

Sugar Snap Peas With Sea Salt Page 120

Wild Mushroom Stroganoff Page 60

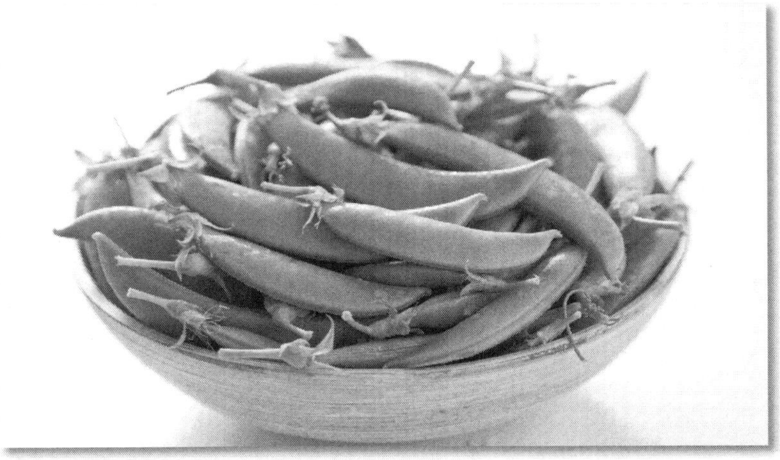

Men's Meal Planner (Eat Little And Often) Week Three

(sc)= slow cooker recipe **(v)** =vegetarian

Men's Meal Planner (Eat Little & Often) 600 Calories Per Fast Day **Week *Three***	
Day One	• **1 Wedge Water Melon** (1/16 of a whole water melon) 88 calories • **Corn & Potato Chowder (sc)** 150 calories • **2 Dutch Crispbakes With 80g Low Fat Cottage Cheese** 120 calories • **Kiwi & Strawberry Smoothie** 100 calories • **Muller Light Yoghurt** 90 calories • **Drinks Throughout The Day** 50 calories *Total calories 598*
Day Two	• **Handful (10) cashew nuts** 100 calories • **¼ Can Tuna With Lemon & tsp Capers + 2 Low Cal Oatcakes** 101 Calories • **Hock Ham & Split Pea Soup (sc)** 178 calories • **18 Plain Pitted Olives** 90 calories • **Dozen whole almonds** 80 calories • **Drinks Throughout The Day** 50 calories *Total calories 599*

Notes: Your shop bought crispbakes should total no more than 60 calories.

Recipe Links:

Corn & Potato Chowder Page 94

Kiwi & Strawberry Smoothie Page 126

Tuna, Lemon & Capers Page 119

Hock Ham & Split Pea Soup Page 98

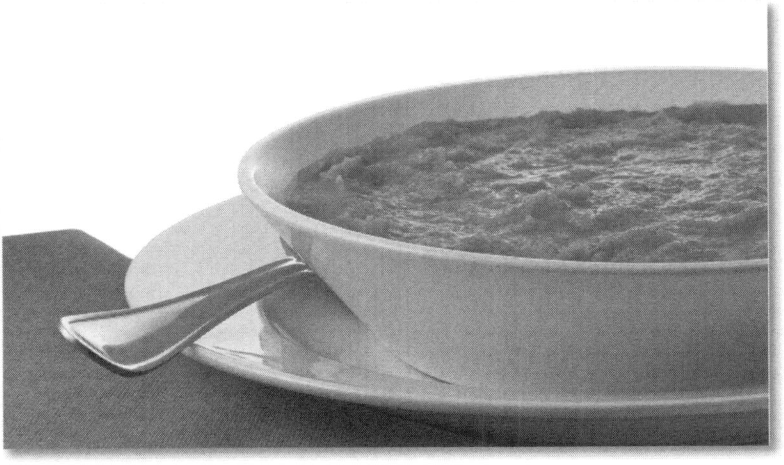

LOW CALORIE 5:2 SLOW COOKER *Recipes*

THE *Skinny* 5:2 DIET SLOW COOKER RECIPE BOOK

Perfect Pulled Pork

Serves 5-6

Calories per serving: 262

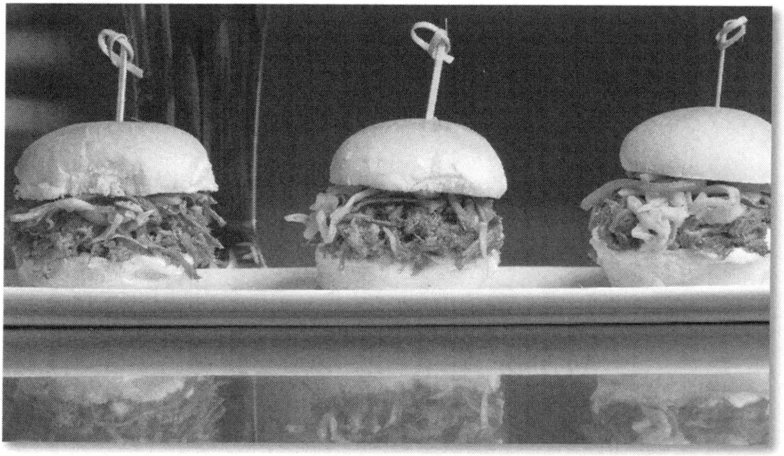

Pulled pork is an absolute classic. It's a chance to use just about everything in your spice rack to create a killer dry rub and it always packs an irresistible punchy and more-ish taste.

Ingredients:

900g/2lb pork butt (shoulder)

1 onion chopped

120ml/ ½ cup BBQ sauce or ketchup

250ml/1 cup beef stock/broth

1 packet BBQ dry rub

Or make your own...

1 tbsp each of garlic powder, brown sugar, onion powder, celery salt, paprika + 1 tsp each mild chilli powder & cumin

Method:

Combine all the spices together and cover the pork in your dry spice rub. Add the stock, onion & BBQ sauce and then place the pork on top. Leave to cook on for 4-6 hours with the lid tightly closed. Ideally you should turn the pork half way through cooking but if you can't don't worry too much. Once the pork is tender enough to fall off the bone remove it from the slow cooker. Leave to rest for as long as you can resist and then use your hands or 2 forks to pull the pork apart. Once it's all shredded, place in a bowl and remove the cooking liquid from the slow cooker. Pour the liquid onto your pork to make beautiful juicy meat.

Family Serving Suggestion (Not 5:2 Followers):

Salad, rolls and barbecue sauce.

Sweet Asian Chicken

Serves 4

Calories per serving: 256

The honey, soy and orange juice in this dish make it a hit with the kids and adds a little eastern flavor to excite evening meal times.

Ingredients:

500g/1lb 2oz skinless chicken breasts

2 garlic cloves crushed

1 onion chopped

60ml/ ¼ cup runny honey

2 tbsp tomato puree/paste

4 tbsp light soy sauce

2 carrots cut into batons

Pinch crushed chilli

120ml/½ cup fresh orange juice

1 tbsp oil

½ tsp cornstarch dissolved in a little water to form a paste

Method:

Combine all the ingredients in a bowl and add to your slow cooker.

Cook on low for 5-6 hours or on high 3-4 hours with the lid tightly shut. Ensure the chicken is cooked through and tender.

Family Serving Suggestion (Not 5:2 Followers):
Fine egg noodles, rice, spring onion and sesame seeds.

Chili Con Carne

Serves 4

Calories per serving: 440

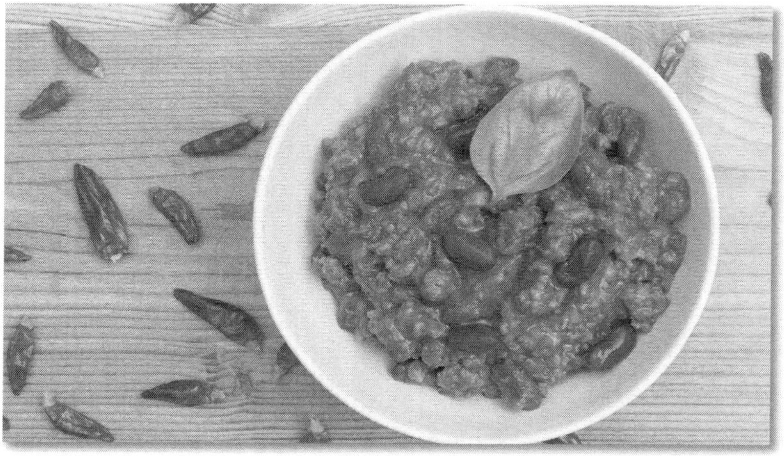

The Spanish name simply means 'chili with meat' and this dish has been a Tex-Mex classic since before the days of the American frontier settlers. Slow cooking the minced beef really allows the flavour to develop and the version here uses the classic kidney bean which is nearly always a hit with the kids.

Ingredients:

550g/1 ¼ lb lean mince/ground beef

1 400g/14oz tin chopped tomatoes

1 400g/14oz tinned kidney beans, drained

1 large onion chopped

1 beef stock cube dissolved into a cup water

500ml/2 cups tomato passata/sieved tomatoes

1 tsp each of brown sugar, oregano, cumin, chili powder, paprika & garlic

½ tsp salt

Method:

Brown the mince and onions in a frying pan. Add all the ingredients into the slow cooker and combine well. Leave to cook on low for 5-6 hours or high 3-4 hours with the lid tightly closed or until the meat is fully cooked.

Family Serving Suggestion (Not 5:2 Followers):
Rice, tortilla chips and a dollop of low fat yoghurt.

Wild Mushroom Stroganoff

Serves 4

Calories Per Serving: 101

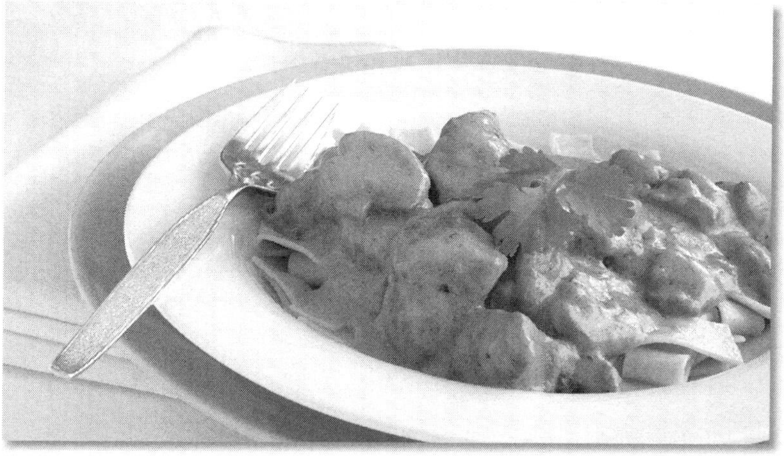

The more exciting the mushrooms the better this dish is going to taste. Use whatever you can get your hands on, a combination of Portobello, Shitake, Morel, Oyster and Enoki would be fantastic, but don't be put off if you can only get regular varieties.

Ingredients:

675g/1 ½ lb wild mixed mushrooms sliced

2 large onions chopped

4 garlic cloves crushed

2 teaspoons smoked paprika

250ml/1 cup vegetable stock

1 400g/14oz tin low fat condensed mushroom soup

Knob butter

Bunch flat chopped leaf parsley (reserve a little for garnish)

Method:

Add all the ingredients into the slow cooker. Close the lid tightly and leave to cook on high for 2-3 hours or low 4-5 hours. Ensure the mushrooms are tender and serve.

Family Serving Suggestion (Not 5:2 Followers):
Pasta or rice.

Italian Meatballs

Serves 5

Calories per serving: 323

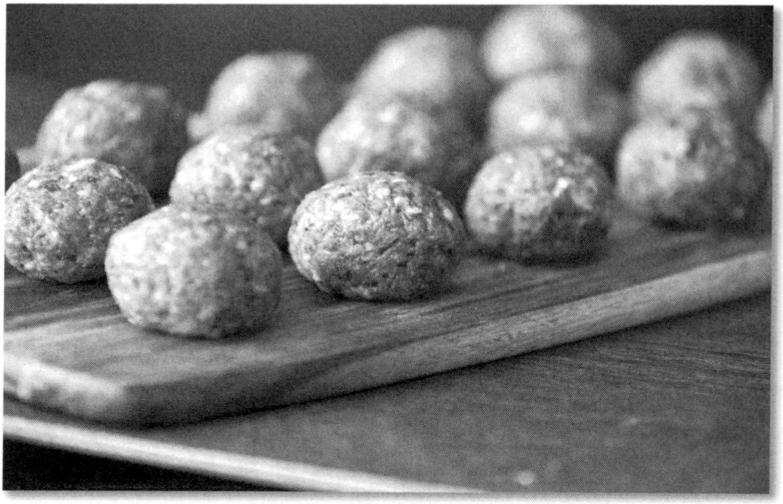

Meatballs are easy to make and never a disappointment to eat. The simple sauce accompanying the meat here is lovely as it is, but a dash of Worcestershire sauce or a tsp of marmite will give it additional depth.

Ingredients:

650g/ 1 ½ lb lean minced/ground beef

1 slice bread whizzed into breadcrumbs

½ onion finely chopped

Handful fresh parsley chopped

1 large egg

1 clove garlic crushed

1 tsp salt

2 400g/14oz tins chopped tomatoes

2 tbsp tomato puree/paste

250ml/1 cup beef stock

1 tsp each of dried basil, oregano & thyme

Method:

Combine together the beef, breadcrumbs, egg, onion, garlic and half the salt. (You can do it with your hands or for super speed put it all into a food mixer).

Once the ingredients are properly mixed together use your hands to shape into about 20-24 meat balls. Add all the ingredients to the slow cooker and combine well. Leave to cook with the lid tightly on for 5-6 hours on low or 3-4 hours on high. Ensure the beef is well cooked and serve.

Family Serving Suggestion (Not 5:2 Followers):
Spaghetti, parmesan cheese and green salad.

Budapest's Best Beef Goulash

Serves 6

Calories per serving: 228

Goulash is a European dish which suits the slow cooker beautifully. After hours of gentle cooking this 'tougher' meat becomes a tender cut which just melts in the mouth.

Ingredients:

900g/2lb lean stewing beef cut into chunks (trim off any fat

1 red (bell) pepper chopped

3 cloves garlic crushed

500 ml/ 2 cups beef stock or boiling water

250ml/ 1 cup red wine

1 400g/14oz tin chopped tomatoes

1 tbsp tomato puree/paste

1 tsp paprika

1 ½ tbsp plain/all purpose flour

1 large onion chopped

Salt & pepper to taste

Method:

Season the beef with salt and pepper and quickly brown in a smoking hot pan. Remove from pan and dust with the flour (the easiest way is to put the cooled beef and flour into a plastic bag and give it a good shake). Add all the ingredients to the slow cooker and combine well. Leave to cook on Low with the lid tightly on for 5-6 hours. Ensure the beef is tender and cooked through, and if you want to thicken it up a little, leave to cook for a further 45 mins with the lid off.

Family Serving Suggestion (Not 5:2 Followers):

Salad and crusty bread or sour cream and tagliatelle pasta.

Enchilada El Salvador

Serves 4
Calories per serving: 324

Inspired by the flavours of Tex Mex this dish is great fun to eat as a family with everyone helping themselves across the table to make their very own perfect enchilada!

Ingredients:

450g/1 lb lean minced/ground beef

1 onion chopped

1 green (bell) pepper chopped

1 400g/14oz tin black beans drained

2 400g/14oz tin chopped tomatoes

250ml/1 cup beef stock/broth

Chilli to taste

4 tsp your favourite packet taco seasoning

Or make your own:

2 tsp mild chilli powder, 1 ½ tsp ground cumin, ½ tsp paprika, ¼ tsp each of onion powder, garlic powder, dried oregano & crushed chilli flakes + 1 tsp each of sea salt & black pepper

Method:

Add all the ingredients to the slow cooker and combine well. Leave to cook with the lid tightly on for 5-6 hours on low or 3-4 hours on high. Ensure the beef is well cooked, if you want to thicken up a little leave to cook for a further 45 mins with the lid off.

Family Serving Suggestion (Not 5:2 Followers):

Flour tortillas, shredded salad, grated cheese and sour cream.

Sweet & Sour Pineapple Pork

Serves 6

Calories per serving: 238

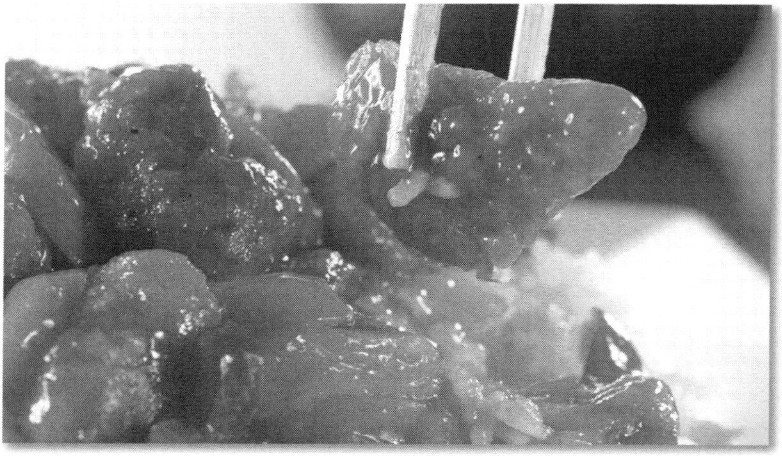

Sweet and Sour is one of the most loved Chinese meals in the world. This is not supposed to be an authentic copy, just take it as a super simple replica which should satisfy your Eastern cravings!

Ingredients:

900g/2lb lean cubed pork

1 tbsp plain/all purpose flour

1 400g/14oz tin pineapple chunks (reserve the juice)

1 onion chopped

1 green (bell) pepper chopped

2 carrots, cut into batons

1 tbsp brown sugar

½ tsp salt

2 tbsp lime juice

1 tbsp light soy sauce

120ml/ ½ cup boiling water

Method:

Brown the pork in a frying pan with a tiny bit of oil. Remove the pork and dust with the flour. Put all the other ingredients except the pineapple chunks into the slow cooker (including the pineapple juice). Combine everything and leave to cook on low for 5-6 hours with the lid tightly closed. Check the pork is tender, add the pineapple chunks and leave for a further 30 min.

Family Serving Suggestion (Not 5:2 Followers):

Boiled rice and prawn crackers.

Sweet & Citrus Salmon

Serves 4

Calories per serving: 270

Like a lot of fresh fish, Salmon can be relatively expensive, so you can substitute for tilapia or basa or talk to your fishmonger for recommendations.

Ingredients:

500g/ 1lb 2oz thick boneless salmon fillets

1 onion chopped

60ml/ ¼ cup light soy sauce

Juice of 2 fresh limes or 4 tbsp lime juice

2 garlic cloves crushed

1 tsp sugar dissolved into 3 tbsp warm water and brushed onto the fillets

Method:

Chop the onion and sauté for a couple of minutes with the garlic in a tiny bit of oil. Remove from the pan and carefully combine all the ingredients in the slow cooker. Cook on low for 1½ hours with the lid tightly on. Check your fish is properly cooked by flaking it a little with a fork.

Family Serving Suggestion (Not 5:2 Followers):

Salad potatoes and carrots.

Best Ever Chicken Curry

Serves 4

Calories per serving: 223

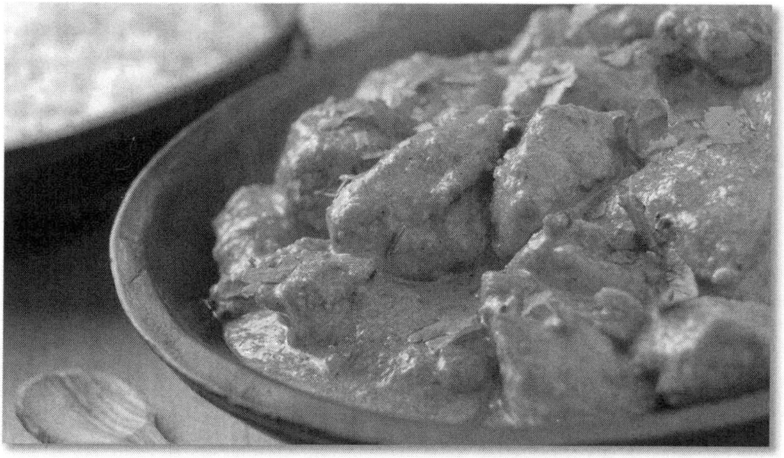

Curry has never been more popular across the world and 'Tikka Masala' is sometimes even referred to as the national dish in the UK! The mix of spices below is preferable, but it's fine to substitute with curry powder if you are in a rush or struggling with store cupboard ingredients.

Ingredients:

500g/1lb 2oz skinless chicken breasts

1 onion chopped

1 tbsp tomato puree

3 cloves garlic crushed

1 tsp low-fat butter spread

375ml/1 ½ cups passata/sieved tomataoes

1 tbsp fresh grated ginger (or use teaspoon of ginger powder)

2 tbsp garam masala

1 tsp ground cumin

1 tsp turmeric

½ tsp chilli powder

or

2 tbsp curry powder is fine (mild works really well with this recipe but use whatever you prefer)

250 ml/1 cup low fat natural yoghurt

Pinch salt

Method:

Combine all your ingredients, except the yoghurt, into your slow cooker. Cook on low for 5-6 hours, or on high 3-4 hours with the lid tightly shut. Ensure the chicken is cooked through and tender, turn off the heat and stir in the yoghurt.

Family Serving Suggestion (Not 5:2 Followers):

Green beans and naan bread.

Hand To Mouth Tex Mex Tacos

Serves 4

Calories Per Serving: 150

Tacos are traditionally eaten with hands not utensils and this gorgeous mix should be no different. Enjoy with friends who don't mind messy eaters!

Ingredients:

1 400g/14oz tin black beans, drained & rinsed

1 400g/14oz tin chopped tomatoes

75g/3oz frozen sweetcorn

1 courgette chopped

1 green (bell) pepper chopped

1 tsp paprika

½ tsp each chilli powder & garlic powder

1 tsp each oregano, thyme, cumin and onion powder

125g/4oz rice

120ml/ ½ cup vegetable stock/broth

Method:

Combine all the ingredients into the slow cooker and cook on low for 5-6 hours with the lid tightly closed or on high 3-4 hours. Check the rice is tender and add more water during cooking if necessary. If you want to thicken the taco mix take the lid off and continue to cook on high for 45 mins or until the consistency is right for you.

Family Serving Suggestion (Not 5:2 Followers):

Taco shells, avocado, lettuce, salsa, cheese, onions and sour cream.

Tuna & Noodle Cattia

Serves 4

Calories per serving: 250

An absolute classic American slow cooker recipe, Tuna & Noodle casserole is always a winner. This version takes it back to basics using the simplest store cupboard ingredients. The title 'Cattia' pays homage to the ancient Latin roots from where the word 'casserole' has its origins.

Ingredients:

350g/12oz fresh egg noodles

1 onion chopped

1 400g/14oz tin fat-free condensed mushroom soup

2 200g/7oz tins tuna steaks or flakes in water

100g/3 ½ oz frozen peas

1 tsp garlic powder

Pinch Salt

Pinch of crushed chilli flakes (if you want a little kick)

Method:

Quickly cook your pasta or noodles in salted boiling water. Save 3 tbsp of the drained water and then combine it along with all the ingredients in the slow cooker and cook on low for 1½ hours.

Family Serving Suggestion (Not 5:2 Followers):

Sliced red onion and tomato salad with parmesan cheese.

Luscious Italian Chicken

Serves 4

Calories per serving: 235

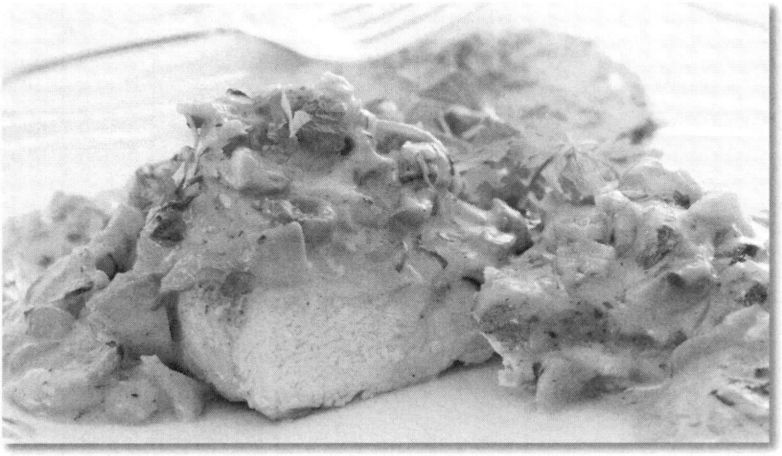

With a lovely creamy consistency this Italian inspired dish makes the most of that wonderful 'cheat' ingredient 'condensed soup'!

Ingredients:

500g/1lb 2oz skinless chicken breasts

2 400g/14oz tins low fat condensed chicken or mushroom soup

100g/3 ½ oz sliced mushrooms

1 onion chopped

Pinch salt

Clove garlic crushed

2 tbsp fat free cream cheese

Dried rub mix of:

1 teaspoon each oregano, rosemary & thyme

Method:

Rub chicken breasts with your dried herb mix and then combine all the ingredients into the slow cooker. Cook on low for 5-6 hours or on high 3-4 hours with the lid tightly shut. Ensure the chicken is cooked through and tender.

Family Serving Suggestion (Not 5:2 Followers):
Vegetables, spaghetti, rice or noodles.

Lean Green Risotto

Serves 4
Calories Per Serving: 285

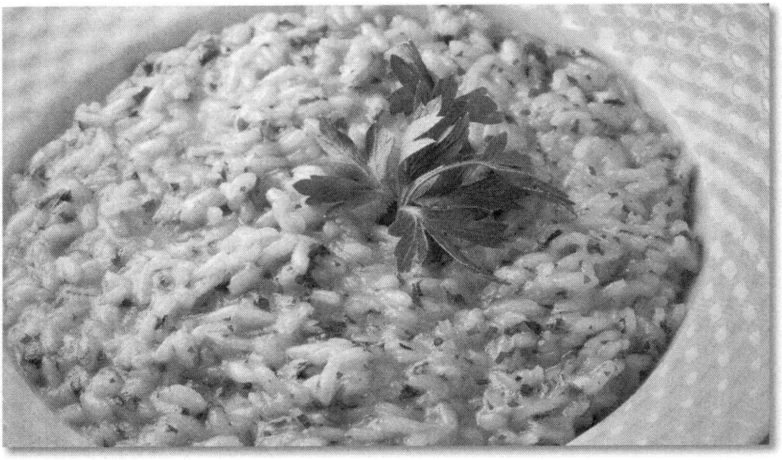

Usually served as a first course in Italy, this veggie pesto version makes a beautiful main course.

Ingredients:

1 tbsp olive oil

Knob butter

1 large onion, chopped

2 cloves of garlic, chopped

225g/8oz risotto rice

1lt/4 cups vegetable stock/broth

1 tsp green pesto

125g/4oz green beans sliced

125g/ 4oz peas

125g/4oz spinach, chopped

Method:

Saute the onion in the oil and butter for a few minutes. Add the risotto to the pan and make sure each grain is coated well with the oil and butter. Transfer to the slow cooker and combine all the ingredients. Leave to cook on High for 2-3 hours with the lid tightly shut, the risotto may need a little more water during cooking so check every half hour or so. Make sure it is cooked to your preference and serve.

Family Serving Suggestion (Not 5:2 Followers):
Basil and rocket salad with parmesan shavings.

Green Thai Fish Curry

Serves 4
Calories per serving: 215

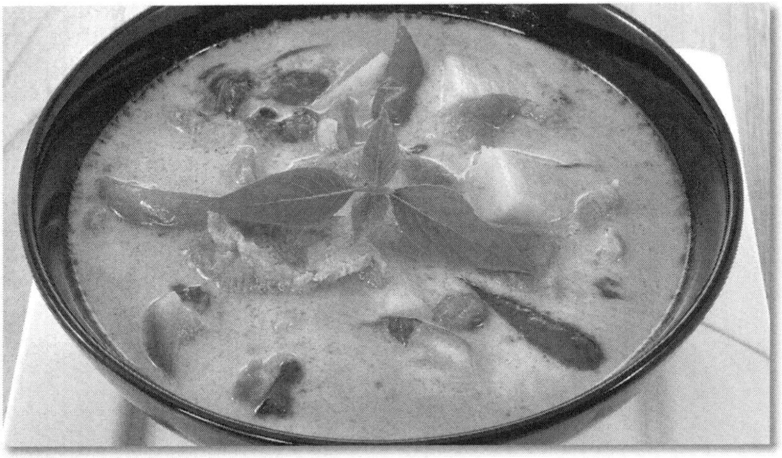

Compared to meat, fish cooks more quickly in the slow cooker and as such fish recipes can be really handy if you haven't got too much cooking time. This recipe is a fantastic and really easy Thai curry which is simple to prep and doesn't take long at all in the slow cooker.

Ingredients:

500g/1 lb 2oz meaty white fish fillets (go for whatever is on sale) haddock, cod, pollock, cobbler... all meaty white fish will work well.

3 small onions chopped

1 tsp fresh ginger or ½ tsp ground ginger

3 cloves garlic crushed

1 whole red chilli

Handful watercress salad

2 tbsp thai green curry paste

250ml/1 cup low fat coconut milk

1 tsp sunflower oil for frying

Pinch salt

Method:

Sauté the onions & green beans with the ginger and garlic over a low heat in a tiny bit of oil. Season the fish fillets with salt and pepper and then carefully combine all the ingredients (except the watercress) in the slow cooker and cook on low for 1 ½ hours with the lid tightly shut. This timing should mean your fish is not over cooked and the green beans have some bite to them. Check your fish is properly cooked through by flaking it a little with a fork and gently add the watercress salad before serving.

If you want to make it a little more aggressive you could add some chopped chili or crushed chilli flakes.

Family Serving Suggestion (Not 5:2 Followers):

Rice or noodles

Slow Spanish Tombet

Serves 4

Calories Per Serving: 115

Tombet is the Spanish version of the French classic ratatouille.

Ingredients:

2 fresh aubergines/eggplant cubed

2 courgettes/zuchinni cut into strips

4 fresh tomatoes cubed

2 peppers, cut into strips

175g/ 6oz tomato puree/paste

2 large red onions, 1 chopped, 1 sliced

1 tsp each of dried marjoram, basil & thyme

½ tsp paprika

1 tsp capers

Handful pitted black olives

3 garlic cloves, crushed

1 tsp each salt & sugar

120ml/ ½ cup vegetable stock/broth

1 tbsp olive oil

Fresh basil to garnish

Method:

Combine all ingredients in the slow cooker and leave to cook on low for 4-5 hours with the lid tightly closed, or on high for 2-3 hours. If you want to thicken the sauce take the lid off and continue to cook on high for 45 mins or until the consistency is right for you.

Family Serving Suggestion (Not 5:2 Followers):

Spanish toast (rough cut farmhouse bread toasted and rubbed with garlic, salt & olive oil).

Zingy Lime Chicken

Serves 4

Calories per serving: 200

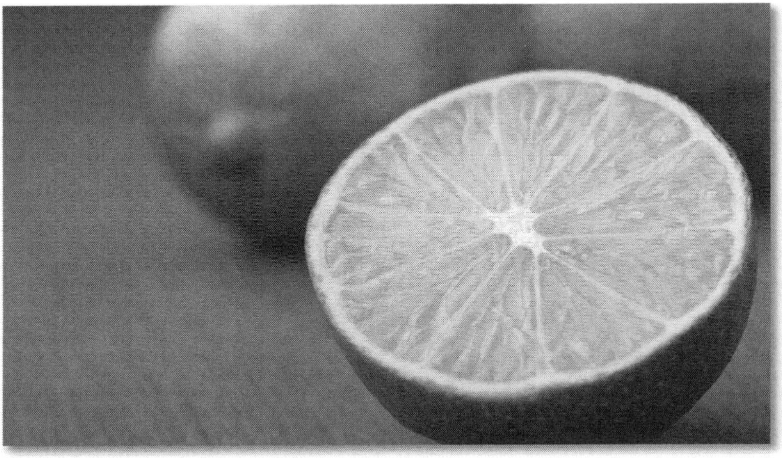

Packed with protein, skinless chicken breasts are a fantastic low-fat meat to use in the slow cooker. The citrus lightness of this recipe is perfect for summer months as well as a welcome taste bud infusion during the cold seasons.

Ingredients:

500g/1lb 2oz skinless large chicken breasts

Juice 2 limes or 3 ½ tablespoons bottled lime juice

Bunch fresh coriander chopped and some to garnish

1 sliced green chilli (or a pinch of dried chilli flakes)

16oz/450g salsa (jar)

Or make your own:

Add 1 onion chopped, 1 clove garlic crushed, 1 green chili chopped to 2 x regular cans (14 oz / 400 g) chopped tomatoes + sea salt to taste

4 tsp your favourite packet taco seasoning

Or make your own:

2 tsp mild chilli powder, 1 ½ tsp ground cumin, ½ tsp paprika, ¼ tsp each of onion powder, garlic powder, dried oregano & crushed chilli flakes + 1 tsp each of sea salt & black pepper

Method:

Put everything together in your slow cooker making sure the chicken is covered with the rest of the ingredients. With the lid tightly shut leave to cook for 4-5 hours on high or 6-8 hours on the low setting. Ensure the chicken is cooked through and tender, then shred it a little with 2 forks.

Family Serving Suggestion (Not 5:2 Followers):

Green salad, rice or quesadillas (flour tortillas).

Shepherd-less Pie

Serves 4
Calories Per Serving 240

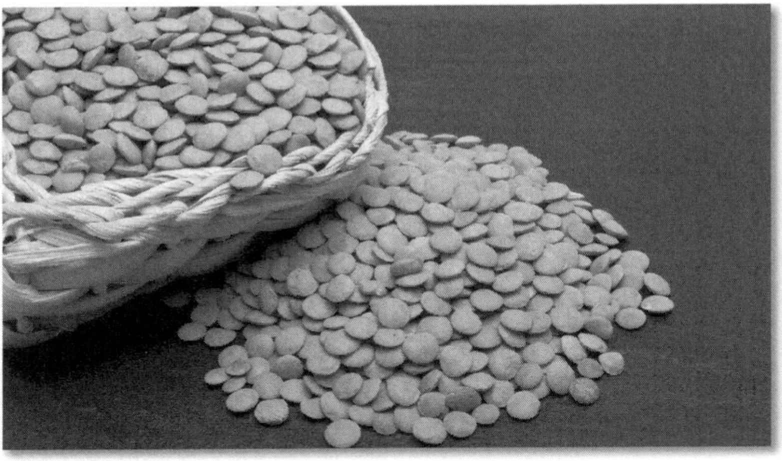

Ingredients:

1 tbsp olive oil

1 onions, chopped

2 carrots, diced

2 stalks celery, chopped

1 garlic cloves, crushed chopped

100g/3 ½ oz mushrooms , sliced

1 bay leaves

1 tsp dried thyme

75g/3oz dried green lentils (soaked overnight)

Splash of red wine if you have it

1 tbsp vegetarian worcestershire sauce

250ml/1 cup vegetable stock/broth

2 tbsp tomato purée/paste

600g/1lb 5oz mashed potato to top the pie

Method:

Gently sauté the onions, celery, carrots and garlic in the herbs for a few minutes. Remove to the slow cooker and combine well with all the other ingredients (except the mashed potato) and leave to cook on low for 4-5 hours with the lid tightly closed, or on high for 2-3 hours. If you want to thicken the sauce take the lid off and continue to cook on high for 45 mins or until the consistency is right for you.

Remove from the slow cooker and place in a oven proof dish. Top with the mashed potato and brown under the grill for a few minutes.

Family Serving Suggestion (Not 5:2 Followers):

Peas and spring greens dressed with garlic oil.

Lovely Lemony Garlicky Chicken

Serves 4

Calories per serving: 208

This is a really simple dish which really benefits from using fresh lemons and fresh basil ideally.

Ingredients:

500g/1lb 2oz skinless chicken breasts

3 garlic cloves crushed

2 whole lemons sliced

1 onion chopped

1 tsp runny honey

1 tsp cornstarch mixed with water to form a paste

500ml/2 cups chicken stock

Salt & pepper to taste

Bunch fresh Basil

Method:

Combine all the ingredients in your slow cooker and leave to cook on low for 5-6 hours or on high 3-4 hours with the lid tightly shut. Ensure the chicken is cooked through and tender.

Family Serving Suggestion (Not 5:2 Followers):

Steamed vegetables and new potatoes.

Slow Cooked Corn On The Cob

Serves 1
Calories 145

Ingredients:

1 medium ear of fresh sweetcorn

1 clove garlic crushed

1 tsp low fat spread

Salt & pepper to taste

Method:

Mix low fat spread and garlic in a bowl, coat the sweetcorn with this mix and wrap in foil. Place in the slow cooker and leave to cook on high with the lid tightly closed for 2 hours or until tender.

St. Patrick's Day Soup

Serves 4

Calories per serving: 100

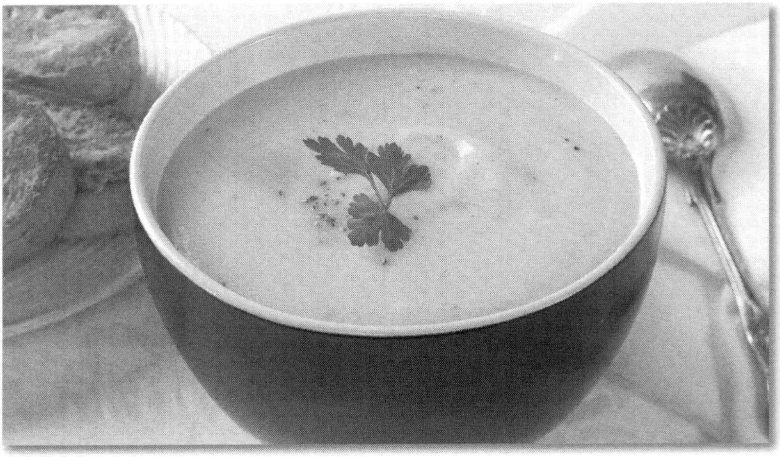

It's often said that everyone is Irish on St. Patrick's day, and here's a chance to get a real taste of Ireland every day with this lovely Irish-inspired potato soup.

Ingredients:

225g/8oz potatoes chopped

1 large onion chopped

3 leeks chopped

Salt & pepper to taste

500ml/2 cups semi skimmed milk

750ml/3 cups vegetable stock/broth

Method:

Combine all the ingredients together in the slow cooker and leave to cook on low for 3-4 hours with the lid tightly shut. Make sure the potatoes are tender, season to taste and then either blend as a smooth soup or eat it rough ready and rustic.

Family Serving Suggestion (Not 5:2 Followers):
Crusty bread, sour cream and chopped parsley.

Corn & Potato Chowder

Serves 4

Calories per serving: 150

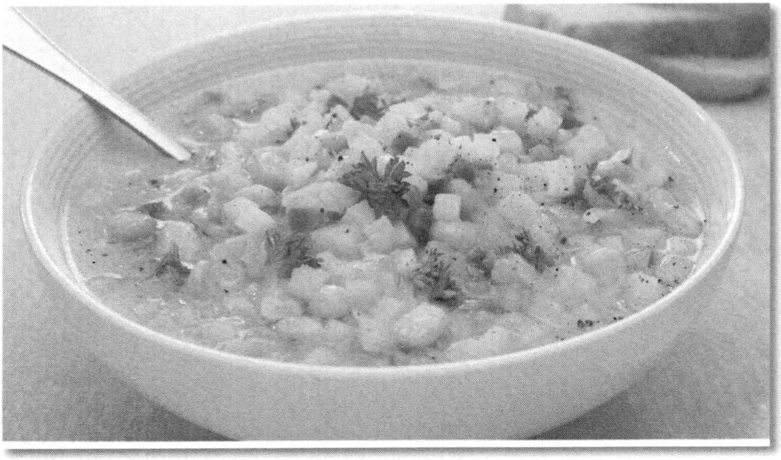

Although primarily associated with seafood, chowder is a lovely thick soup recipe which works just as well with vegetables alone. You could easily add some smoked haddock to this recipe if you wanted to be authentic, but this veggie option is good too.

Ingredients:

1 onion chopped

400g/14oz sweetcorn

1 400g/14oz tin creamed sweetcorn

2 cloves garlic crushed

750 ml/3 cups vegetable stock

175g/6oz potatoes diced

1 tsp low fat butter spread

500/2 cups semi skimmed milk

1 tsp salt

Method:

Sauté the onion and garlic in a tiny bit of oil. Place all the ingredients in the slow cooker and cook on low for 3-4 hours with the lid tightly shut. Ensure the potatoes are tender and mash a little with a fork to create the right consistency.

Family Serving Suggestion (Not 5:2 Followers):

Saltine or cream crackers.

Super Simple Chicken Taco Soup

Serves 4-6

Calories per serving: 247

No one knows when Taco turned into soup, but whenever it was it's a firm favourite which is worth celebrating in the slow cooker.

Ingredients:

125g/4oz skinless chicken breast

400g/14oz sweet corn

1 400g/14oz tin black beans

1 400g/14oz tin kidney beans

1 400g/14oz tin chopped tomatoes

2 cloves garlic minced

1lt/4 cups warm water

1 chilli chopped or a pinch of dried crushed chilli flakes (add as much as you like)

4 tsp your favourite packet taco seasoning

Or make your own

2 tsp mild chilli powder, 1 ½ tsp ground cumin, ½ tsp paprika, ¼ tsp each of onion powder, garlic

powder, dried oregano & crushed chilli flakes + 1 tsp each of sea salt & black pepper

Method:

Season your chicken breast and place at the bottom of the slow cooker. Add all the other ingredients and leave to cook for 2 hours on high or 3 hours on low with the lid tightly shut. Ensure the chicken is cooked through and tender, then shred it a little with 2 forks through the soup.

If you want to thicken the soup up at all after cooking, take the lid off and cook on high for a further 45minutes or until you get the consistency you want.

Family Serving Suggestion (Not 5:2 Followers):

Tortilla chips, crusty bread or over rice.

Hock Ham & Split Pea Soup

Serves 4
Calories per serving: 178

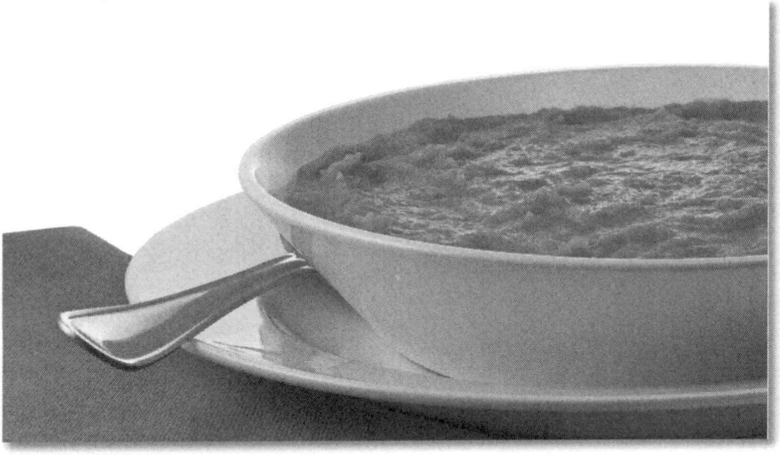

Ham hocks are a bargain ingredient that can give a real depth to a dish. You could substitute ham hocks for a meaty ham bone if you had one left after a family gathering.

Ingredients:

2 ham knuckles (if you can buy them smoked, even better)

3 carrots

2 celery stalks

1 onion chopped

3 garlic cloves

450g/1lb green split peas (yellow or green are fine)

1 ½ lt/5 cups warm water

Method:

Combine all the ingredients into the slow cooker and cook on low for 7-8 hours or high for 4-5 hours with the lid tightly shut. When the soup is cooked take out the hocks and strip the meat, if they are fully cooked the meat should fall away easily. Get rid of any fat and stir the shredded ham back into the soup. If you want to alter the texture you can thicken it up by mashing the split peas a little before putting the ham meat back in.

Asian Hot Soup

Serves 4

Calories Per Serving: 130

This is a lovely version of Chinese Hot & Sour soup, which is believed to be good for colds, so feel free to load up on the fresh ginger if you can handle it.

Ingredients:

50g/2oz shiitake mushrooms

50g/2oz cloud ear fungus (if you can get them or closed cap if you can't)

200g/7oz tinned bamboo shoots, drained

3 cloves garlic, crushed

1 tsp sesame oil

1 tsp chilli paste (or dried crushed chilies to taste)

2 tbsp rice wine vinegar or wine vinegar

225g/8oz frozen peas

2 tbsp soy sauce

1 tsp sesame oil

275g/10oz tofu, cubed

1 tbsp freshly grated ginger

750ml/3 cups vegetable stock

Method:

Combine all the ingredients in your slow cooker and leave to cook of low 5-6 hours with the lid tightly shut or high for 3-4 hours.

Zucchini Soup

Serves 4
Calories Per Serving: 95

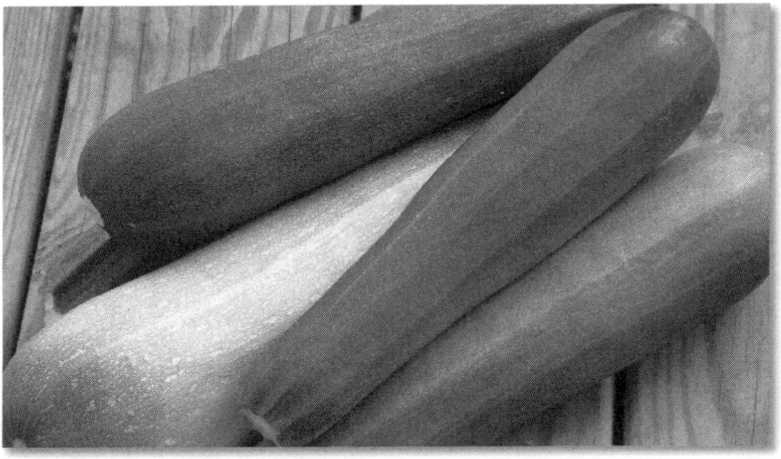

You can mix this soup up by switching the broccoli and courgette measurements during cooking.

Ingredients:

75g/3oz potatoes, cubed

1 lt/4 cups vegetable stock

1 head broccoli, chopped

1 head cauliflower, chopped

1 tsp each cumin and paprika

Salt to taste

1 tsp olive oil

1 onion

2 garlic cloves, crushed

3 courgettes/zuchinni chopped

Method:

Gently sauté the onion and courgettes in the oil for a couple of minutes. Add all the ingredients into the slow cooker and leave to cook on low for 5-6 hours or high for 3-4 hours with the lid tightly shut.

Blend to get the required consistency.

Family Serving Suggestion (Not 5:2 Followers):

Swirl of fresh cream, parmesan and some crumbled stilton cheese.

Barley & Chestnut Mushroom Soup

Serves 4

Calories Per Serving: 175

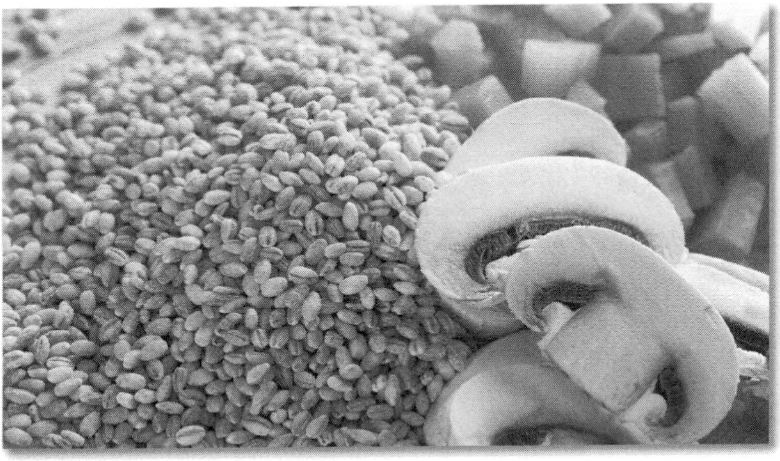

This is a really tasty and filling soup. The mushrooms should be finely chopped to give the soup some body.

Ingredients:

1 large onion, chopped

1 tsp olive oil

1 carrot chopped

1 celery stalk, chopped

200g/7oz mushrooms finely chopped

1 400g/14oz tin chopped tomatoes

200g/7oz frozen sweet corn

75g/3oz pearl barley

1 tsp each of basil, oregano, thyme

Salt & Pepper to taste

3 cloves garlic, crushed

1 ¼ lt/5 cups vegetable stock

Method:

Gently sauté the onions, carrot, mushrooms and celery in a frying pan with the oil for a few minutes then combine all the ingredients into the slow cooker and cook on low for 5-6 hours with the lid tightly closed or on high 3-4 hours.

Bean, Rosemary and Roasted Garlic Dip

Serves 12-14
Calories Per Serving: 88

Ingredients:

6 garlic cloves chopped

100g/3 ½ oz parmesan cheese grated

1 bunch chopped fresh rosemary

2 tbsp extra virgin olive oil

1 400g/14oz tin borlotti beans drained

125g/4oz low fat cream cheese

Handful chopped black olives

1 tbsp white wine vinegar

250ml/1 cup water

1 tbsp lemon juice

Salt to taste

Method:

Quickly pulse all the ingredients (except the lemon juice) in a food processor. Empty the blitzed mixture into the slow cooker and leave to cook on low for 1-2 hours. If the mixture it too thick add a little more water. If it's not thick enough continue to cook with the lid off until you get the required consistency. After cooking allow to cool and stir in the lemon juice.

Family Serving Suggestion (Not 5:2 Followers):

Raw celery, cucumber and carrot batons.

Nacho Bean & Onion Dip

Serves 10-12
Calories per serving: 90

Ingredients:

2 400g/14oz tins low fat refried beans

1 fresh green chilli finely chopped

250ml/1 cup water

1 large onion chopped

100g/3 ½ oz mozzarella cheese chopped

1 packet of your favourite taco seasoning mix

Or make your own:

2 tsp mild chilli powder, 1 ½ tsp ground cumin, ½ tsp paprika, ¼ tsp each of onion powder, garlic powder, dried oregano & crushed chilli flakes + 1 tsp each of sea salt & black pepper

Salt to taste

1 tbsp lemon juice

Method:

Place all the ingredients, except the lemon juice, into the slow cooker and combine well. Leave to cook on low for 1-2 hours. If the mixture it too thick add a little more water. If it's not thick enough continue to cook with the lid off until you get the required consistency. Stir in the lemon juice before serving.

Family Serving Suggestion (Not 5:2 Followers):
Tortilla chips or breadsticks.

Multi Grain Breakfast

Serves 4
Calories Per Serving: 225

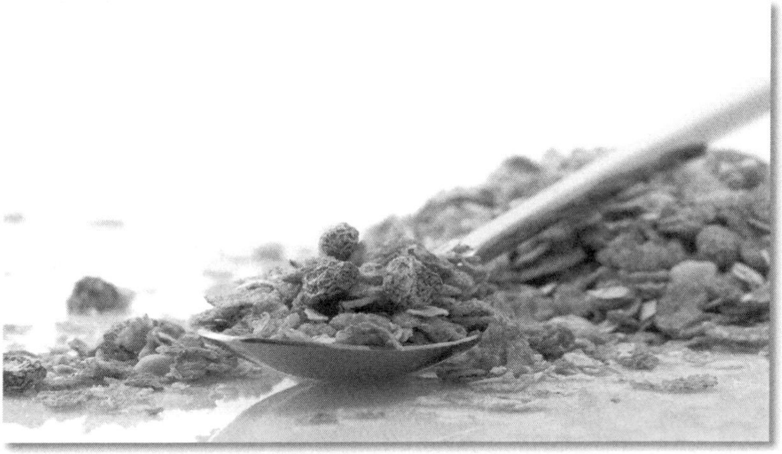

This is a lovely way to start your day. Just load up your slow cooker in the evening and leave to cook overnight.

Ingredients:

25g/1oz rolled oats

75g/3 oz bulgur wheat

100g/3 ½ oz brown rice

25g/1 oz pearl barley

50g/2oz quinoa

150g/5oz chopped apple (no need to peel)

75g/3oz raisins

1 tsp ground cinnamon

1 tbsp vanilla extract

750ml/3 cups water

Sprinkle of nutmeg

Method:

Combine all the ingredients (except the nutmeg) well in the slow cooker and leave to cook overnight on low for 6 to 8 hours with the lid tightly shut. Add more water during cooking if needed and stir well. Sprinkle with nutmeg after cooking.

Family Serving Suggestion (Not 5:2 Followers):
Add vanilla soymilk and organic maple syrup to your taste.

Morning Millet

Serves 8

Calories per serving 155

It's best to cook up a large batch of this which the family can share or you can store in the fridge.

Ingredients:

250g/9oz millet

750 ml/3 cups vanilla rice milk

3 apples, peeled, cored and chopped

¼ tsp

Method:

Combine all ingredients in the slow cooker and cook on high for 4 hours or on low for 8 hours with the lid tightly shut. Add water if needed to loosen the mixture during cooking.

SIMPLE LOW CALORIE 5:2 BREAKFAST, SNACK & LUNCH *Recipes*

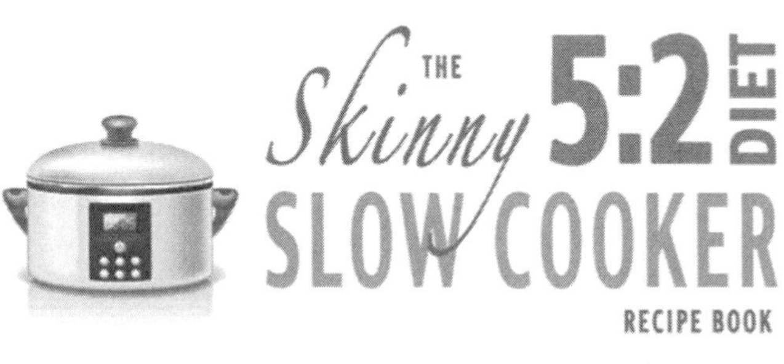

Muesli

Serves 10
124 calories per serving

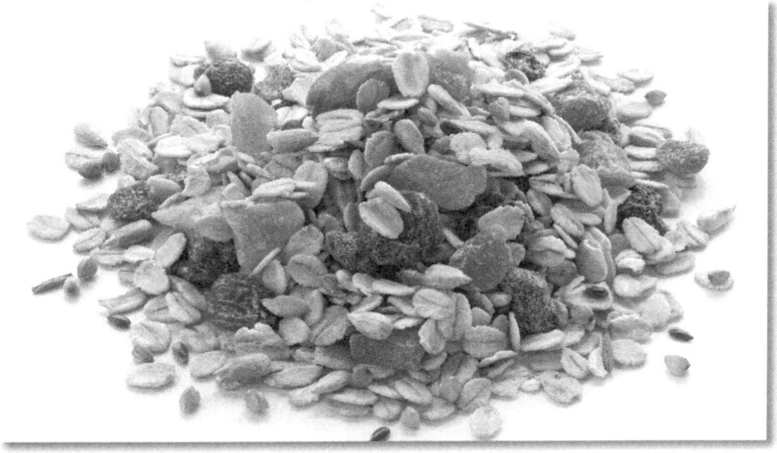

Ingredients:

175g/6oz jumbo oats

600g/1lb 5oz Allbran

15g/ ½ oz wheatgerm

50g/2oz raisins

75g/3 oz ready-to-eat apricots, chopped

50g/2 oz golden linseeds

Method:

Combine all ingredients together and serve with skimmed milk.

Fruit Salad

Serves 3
Calories per serving 138

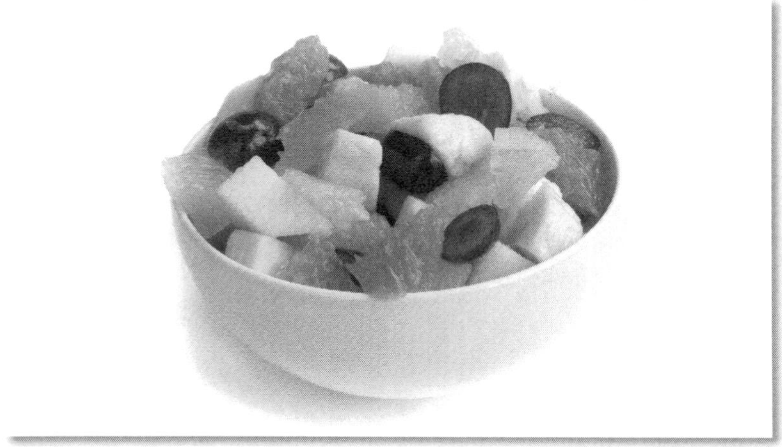

Ingredients:

1 large orange

1 large apple

1 small banana

225g/8oz seedless grapes

1 tsp brown sugar

Method:

Chop all the fruit and sprinkle with sugar

Tuna & Pitta Salad

Serves 1
Calories 260

Ingredients:

50g/2oz tinned tuna (in water)

2 tsp low fat mayonnaise

1 whole wheat pitta bread

25g/1oz spinach

1 tsp lemon juice

2 spring onions chopped

Method:

Combine all ingredients together (except pitta) and stuff inside the pitta bread.

Carrot & Celery Salad

Serves 1
Calories 97

Ingredients

2 peeled grated carrots

1 lemon, juiced

1 stalk celery, chopped

1 slice tinned pineapple

Pinch of salt

Method:

Combine all ingredients well in a bowl.

Grilled Chicken & Tomato Snack

Serves 1
Calories 100

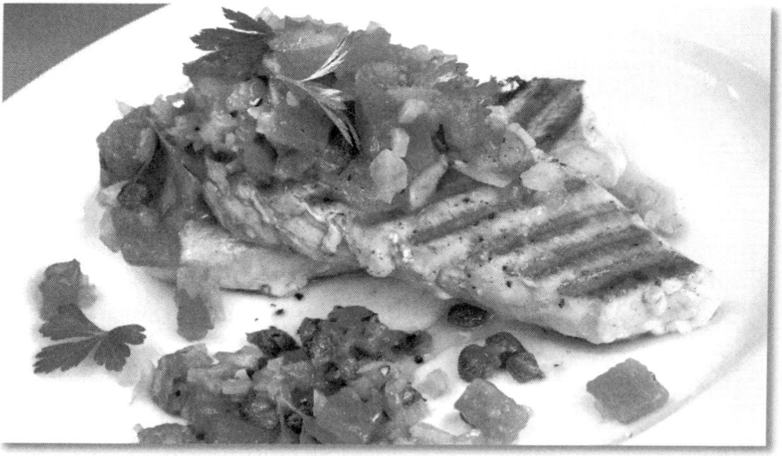

Ingredients:

75g/3oz chicken breast

150g/5oz ripe cherry tomatoes, halved

Method:

Season with plenty of salt and pepper and place your half chicken breast and cherry tomatoes under the grill and leave to cook on a medium heat for 8 minutes each side (or until the chicken is thoroughly cooked). Add some fresh basil or flat leaf parsley to garnish.

Tuna, Lemon & Capers

Serves 1
Calories 100

Ingredients

50g/2 oz tinned tuna (in water)

Squeeze of lemon juice

1 tsp capers, finely chopped

2 low cal oat cakes

Method:

Combine tuna, capers and lemon juice together and serve on top of oatcakes.

Sugar Snap Peas With Sea Salt

Serves 1

Calories 65

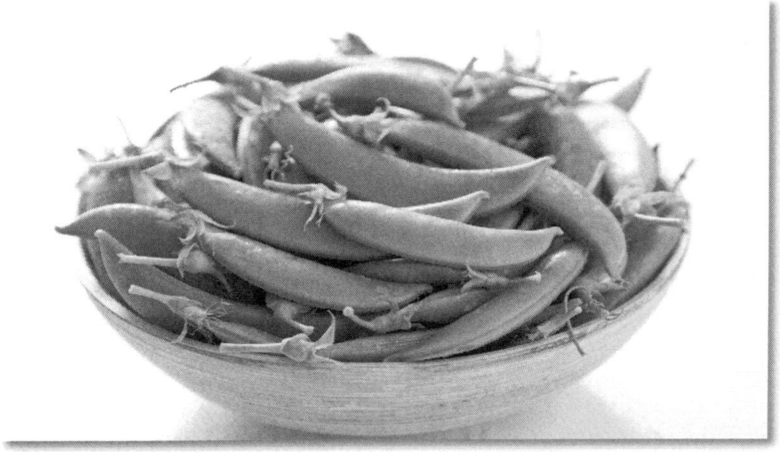

Ingredients:

100g/3 ½ oz sugar snap peas

1 tsp low fat spread

1 tsp crushed sea salt

1 tsp chopped fresh mint or basil

Method:

Place peas in a pan of boiling water for 1 minute, drain and then add spread & herbs into pan. When spread has melted through the peas transfer to bowl and sprinkle with sea salt.

Homemade Salsa

Serves 1
Calories 65

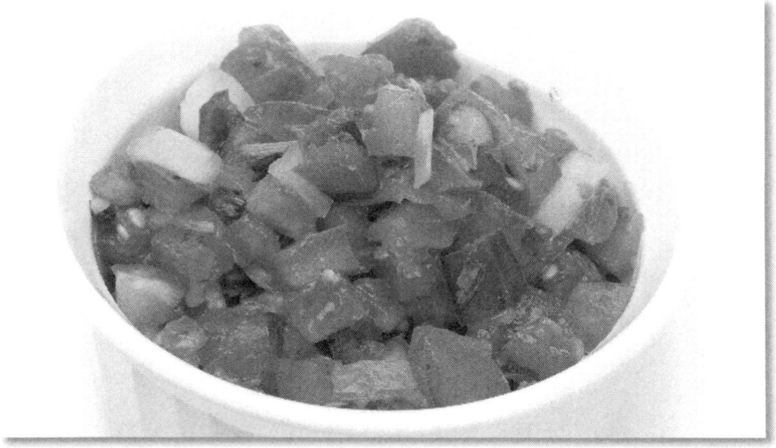

Ingredients:

125g/4oz fresh tomatoes, finely chopped

½ onion, finely chopped

1 green chillies, finely chopped

Small bunch fresh coriander, finely chopped

salt, to taste

lime juice, to taste

1 tbsp water

Method:

Combine all ingredients together. Can be stored in airtight container for several days and used to liven up many meals and snacks.

Tomato, Olive & Feta Salad

Serves 1
Calories 113

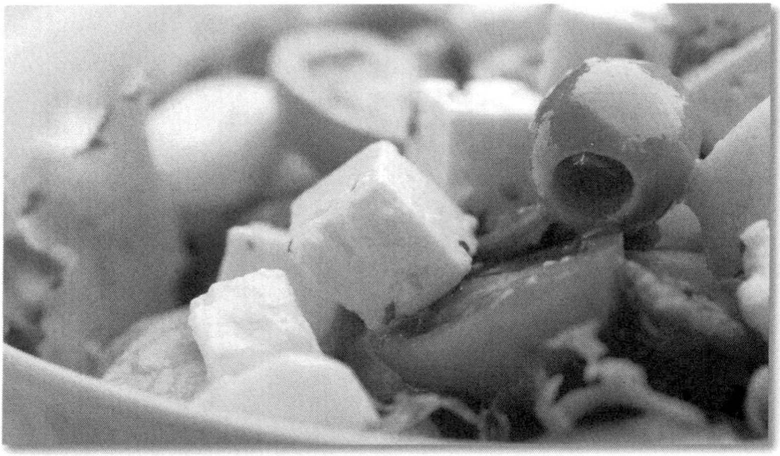

Ingredients:

2 medium tomatoes sliced

Seasonal salad leaves

1 tsp olive oil

25g/1 oz low fat feta cheese, crumbled

1 tsp fresh basil, chopped

Splash red wine vinegar

1 garlic cloves crushed

5 pitted olives

Method:

Combine all ingredients well in a bowl.

Cauliflower Rice

Serves 4
Calories per serving 50

Ingredients:

1 large head cauliflower

Method:

Whizz a whole head of cauliflower in the food processor until the pieces are a size of a grain of rice.

Microwave it in a covered dish for 5-7 minutes and use as substitute for regular rice.

Freeze any leftovers in portions.

Strawberry & Banana Smoothie

Serves 1
Calories 100

Ingredients

250ml/1 cup fat free Greek yoghurt

1/2 large banana

3 large strawberries

Handful of ice

Method:

Add yoghurt to blender followed by other ingredients. You can use frozen or fresh fruit. Blend until smooth, add ice to get your preferred consistency.

Mixed Berry Smoothie

Serves 1
Calories 100

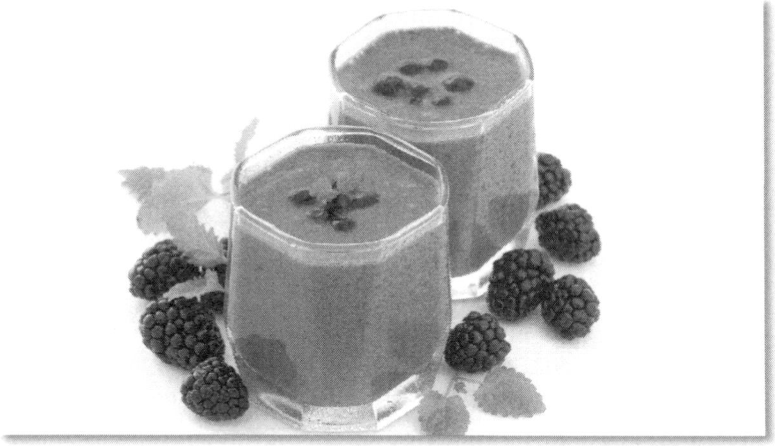

Ingredients:

1 banana

250g/9oz mixed fruit berries - raspberries, blueberries, blackberries

250ml/1 cup fat free Greek yoghurt

Handful of ice

Method:

Add yoghurt to blender followed by other ingredients. You can use frozen or fresh fruit. Blend until smooth, add ice to get your preferred consistency.

Kiwi & Strawberry Smoothie

Serves 1
Calories 100

Ingredients:

1 banana

1 kiwi fruit

5 strawberries

1 teaspoon Agave nectar

120ml/ ½ cup skimmed milk

3 Handfuls of ice

Method:

Add all the ingredients to the blender. You can use frozen or fresh fruit.

Blend until smooth, add ice to get your preferred consistency.

Please give us your feedback

We'd love to hear about your 5:2 diet experience so feel free to leave a review. Reviews help others decide if this is the right book for them so a moment of your time would be very welcome. Thank you.

You may also be interested in other titles in the CookNation series:

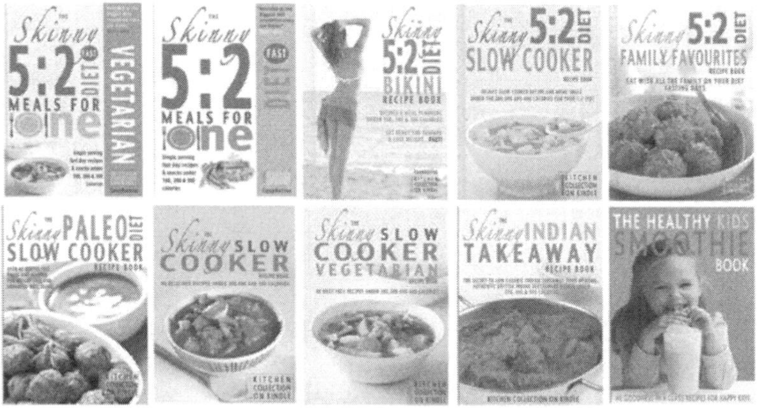

The Skinny 5:2 Fast Diet Vegetarian Meals For One
Single Serving Fast Day Recipes & Snacks Under 100, 200 & 300 Calories.

The Skinny 5:2 Fast Diet Meals For One
Single Serving Fast Day Recipes & Snacks Under 100, 200 & 300 Calories.

The Skinny 5:2 Bikini Diet Recipe Book
Recipes & Meal Planners Under 100, 200 & 300 Calories. Get Ready For Summer & Lose Weight... FAST!
The Skinny 5:2 Family Favourites Recipe Book
(UK & US Editions)
Eat With All the Family On Your Diet Fasting Days.

The Skinny Slow Cooker Recipe Book
40 Delicious Recipes Under 300, 400 And 500 Calories.

The Skinny Slow Cooker Vegetarian Recipe Book
40 Delicious Recipes Under 200, 300 And 400 Calories.

The Skinny Paleo Diet Slow Cooker Recipe Book
Over 40 Gluten Free Paleo Diet Recipes For Weight Loss And Enhanced Well Being.

The Skinny Indian Takeaway Recipe Book
Authentic British Indian Restaurant Dishes Under 300, 400 And 500 Calories.

The Healthy Kids Smoothie Book
40 Delicious Goodness In A Glass Recipes for Happy Kids.

Find all these great titles by searching under **'CookNation'** on **Amazon**.

Conversion Chart

Weights for dry ingredients

Metric	Imperial
7g	¼ oz
15g	½ oz
20g	¾ oz
25g	1 oz
40g	1½oz
50g	2oz
60g	2½oz
75g	3oz
100g	3½oz
125g	4oz
140g	4½oz
150g	5oz
165g	5½oz
175g	6oz
200g	7oz
225g	8oz
250g	9oz
275g	10oz
300g	11oz
350g	12oz
375g	13oz
400g	14oz
425g	15oz
450g	1lb
500g	1lb 2oz
550g	1¼lb
600g	1lb 5oz
650g	1lb 7oz
675g	1½lb
700g	1lb 9oz

Metric	Imperial
750g	1lb 11oz
800g	1¾lb
900g	2lb
1kg	2¼lb
1.1kg	2½lb
1.25kg	2¾lb
1.35kg	3lb
1.5kg	3lb 6oz
1.8kg	4lb
2kg	4½lb
2.25kg	5lb
2.5kg	5½lb
2.75kg	6lb

Liquid measures

Metric	Imperial	Aus	US
25ml	1fl oz		
60ml	2fl oz	¼ cup	¼ cup
75ml	3fl oz		
100ml	3½fl oz		
120ml	4fl oz	½ cup	½ cup
150ml	5fl oz		
175ml	6fl oz	¾ cup	¾ cup
200ml	7fl oz		
250ml	8fl oz	1 cup	1 cup
300ml	10fl oz/½ pt	1¼ cups	
360ml	12fl oz		
400ml	14fl oz		
450ml	15fl oz	2 cups	2 cups/1 pint
600ml	1 pint	1 pint	2½ cups
750ml	1¼ pint		
900ml	1½ pints		
1 litre	1¾ pints	1/34 pints	1 quart

7713070R00072

Made in the USA
San Bernardino, CA
15 January 2014